Sharon

— Chappy Chanukah
1990

DISEASES AND THERAPEUTICS
OF THE SKIN

...and any time you
want to look at my
psoriasis, you only
have to ask....

DISEASES AND THERAPEUTICS OF THE SKIN

BY

J. HENRY ALLEN, M. D.

PROFESSOR OF SKIN AND VENEREAL DISEASES,
HERING MEDICAL COLLEGE,
CHICAGO, ILL.

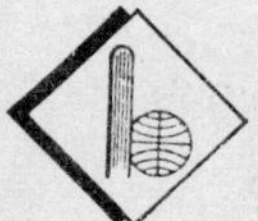

B. Jain Publishers Pvt. Ltd.
New Delhi (India)

Price : Rs. 20.00

Reprint Edition : 1990
© Copyright with the Publisher
Published by :
B. Jain Publishers Pvt. Ltd.
1921, Street No. 10, Chuna Mandi
Paharganj, New Delhi - 110 055 (INDIA)
Printed at :
J. J. Offset Printers
Kishan Kunj, Delhi - 110 092

ISBN 81—7021—054—2
BOOK CODE B-2007

DEDICATION

I dedicate this little work to one to whom I am not only indebted for my recovery from a severe illness that seemed impossible to me, but who was one of the first to arouse in me the importance of following Hahnemann's principles; who has ever been one of the most ardent and faithful followers of true Homœopathy, whose wise counsel in many cases has shown me the depth of his knowledge of the law of similars. That Homœopathy might boast of many more such physicians as Dr. J. R. Haynes of Indiánapolis, Indiana, is my sincere wish.

J. HENRY ALLEN, M.D.

PREFACE

In the preparation of this little work we have endeavored to present this very difficult subject in as clear and as concise a manner as possible, leaving out all unnecessary detail that might in any way confuse or burden the mind of the busy practitioner or student of dermatology. It is our wish to make it one of practical use to the busy practitioner as well as a text-book for the student who wishes to receive a practical knowledge of this subject, avoiding as much as possible the unnecessary task of reading voluminous works written by noted specialists upon the subject. The history, pathology and pathological anatomy has been dealt with briefly, partially owing to the present uncertain knowledge on these subjects, and partially to the differences of opinion held by the homœopathic physician and our colleague of the regular school. We also have endeavored to make the therapeutic part as strong as possible, limited as we are by lack of space in a work of this size, hoping later on to materially strengthen it by a repertory wholly confined to the subject. The homœopathics of diseases of the skin have by no means been forgotten, as we feel that Homœopathy can be as fully and as ably demonstrated through the law of similia, by the homœopathic physician in the dermatological field, as has been in the past in any other department of medicine. We feel greatly indebted to the many strong and able writers upon this subject, such as Drs. Morrow, Fox, Shoemaker, Hyde and others, whose valuable assistance has aided much in the production of the work.

THE AUTHOR

PREFACE TO THE FIRST INDIAN EDITION

The reprinting of Dr. Allen's DISEASES AND THERA-PEUTICS OF THE SKIN gives to the Homœopathic practitioner something he has sorely needed, something his homœopathic brethren have had for many years; a book which gives the description, etiology, diagnosis and treatment according to the law of similars. The readers will know how to keep a good skin. That Skin's diseases are for the most part diseases of the constitution and not diseases of the cutaneous surface alone, has been clearly proved in this book. We hope it will be welcome information to the profession.

PUBLISHER

TABLE OF CONTENTS

PART I

PART III

PART IV

PART V

PART VI

PART VII

PART VIII

Classification—Parasites, Vegetable

Animal Parasites

PART IX

Dermatological Therapeutics

DISEASES OF THE SKIN

PART I

GENERAL ANATOMY AND PHYSIOLOGY

The study of Pathology is a study of the structure of a tissue or organ, when it has undergone changes due to disease, as compared with a healthy or normal tissue as a standard. So, in the study of the skin, no exception can be made to this rule, hence, a comprehensive knowledge of its Anatomy and Physiology is necessary in order to fully understand the manifold changes that take place within its structure.

In the many classifications of the diseases we meet we frequently find, in each, some special tissues involved, and again a number may be involved. It is, therefore, evident that a study of the normal structures of the skin will materially aid us in the appreciation of its diseases.

The *integumentum commune* forms an external covering for the whole organism and is intimately situated to the structure lying beneath it, and continuous with the mucous membrane at the natural orifices. It is firm, fibrous, elastic, its color varying with the age, sex, race, and climate. It is thickest on the back, buttocks, palms of the hands and soles of the feet, thinnest on the eyelids and prepuce.

The surface of the skin is not smooth, but shows greater or lesser elevations and depressions, due to the presence of furrows or grooves, which divide the whole surface into oblong or quadrilateral shaped spaces, seen more distinctly about the joints and the flexures of the body, their direction being in the direction of the greatest tension of the skin.

The pores correspond to the openings of the hair follicles, the sebaceous and sweat glands. Hairs are present all over the body, except on palms of the hands and soles of the feet, the last phalanges of the fingers and toes, glans penis and inner surface of prepuce. The smaller or almost invisible hairs are called lanugo.

The skin is commonly divided into three layers: First, Epidermic; second, Corium, Derma, or Cutis Vera, with the papillæ; third, subcutaneous connective tissues with its adipose. The bloodvessels and lymphatics are situated in the latter two layers. The nerves are distributed to all three layers except the uppermost layer of the epidermis, known as the scarf skin. The appendages of the skin are sudoriferous or sweat glands, sebaceous glands, hairs and nails.

MINUTE ANATOMY

The minute anatomy and the histological elements of these different layers may be briefly considered, first taking up the Epidermis or Epithelial layer. It is a laminated, slightly elastic membrane composed wholly of epithelial cells and scales containing no bloodvessels, with a very scant supply of nerves, just a few filaments. It covers the corium, everywhere protecting it from external injury or irritation, pierced by the hair follicles, the sweat and sebaceous glands; it is marked as before mentioned by a network of minute furrows which represent the depressions between the papillæ. The epidermis consists of four separate layers: First, Stratum Corium; second, Stratum Lucidum; third, Stratum Granulosum; fourth, Stratum Mucosum. The first two layers are considered together as the horny layer and the latter two as the mucous layer, but in our pathological study of the skin it is necessary to study the four separate layers, on account of their separate and special involvement in the different diseases we meet.

Stratum Corium, the external layer, is composed of several layers of flat scales or epithelia, free from nuclei or granulations; they desquamate all through life, and their mode of growth is not yet settled.

Stratum Lucidum is a thin layer quite transparent (hence its name) lying directly beneath the corium layer. It consists of from four to six rows of staff-shaped cells, with flattened nuclei. It is frequently called the stratum of Oehl.

Stratum Granulosum consists of two or three rows of flattened nucleated cells, somewhat spindle shaped, granular around their nuclei. These granulations are supposed to be a substance intermediate in nature between protoplasm and keratin.

One author believes the color of the skin in the white race depends on those granules, and that the stratum lucidum is developed from them, as they have the power to strongly refract the light.

Stratum Mucosum, Stratum Malpighii or Rete Mucosum; this layer lies immediately above the corium, separated from it by a thin membrane. It adapts itself into the papillary layer of the corium by means of an inter-papillary arrangement which fits into the depressions, composed of several layers of nucleated cells, varying in size and shape. The first few layers are columnar, with oval shaped nuclei, arranged with their large axis perpendicular to the surface of the corium. The lower layers of cells are cubiform, polygonal, with special nuclei; homogeneous in their structure, enclosed in a cell wall, and contain granular pigmentary matter.

The cells of the superficial strata are larger and more granular and become flattened as they approach the surface. The color of this layer is from a yellowish tinge to a brown or black, depending on the race.

The Corium, Derma or Cutis Vera is the most interesting layer for study, as it is the most highly organized portion of the skin. It is composed of white fibrous connective tissue, arranged in bundles, interspersed with a muscular element, and yellow elastic fibres, lymphoid corpuscles, fat globules, as well as true connective tissue cells, are found within the closely interwoven spaces. The average thickness is from 1.69 to 2.26 m.m., of course much thicker on the parts before mentioned. The Corium contains nerves, lymphatics, hairs, glands. It is divided into two layers, the upper and lower. The outer layer is called Pars-Papillaris or papillary layer, and the inner layer Pars-Reticularis. The number of these little papillæ that cover the entire surface of the body are estimated by Sappey to be 150,000,000. These papillæ are of two varieties, the vascular and the nervous; they contain the terminal loops of the bloodvessels and nerves.

Pars-Reticularis—This layer is the fibrous and connective tissue layer forming the bulk of the cutis. The history of its development in embryonic life is wonderfully interesting. (See Morrow, Vol. III., p. 9.)

Subcutaneous tissue is made up of connective tissue bundles crossing each other and interlacing in such a way as to form rhomboid spaces. These spaces contain fat globules arranged in lobes separated by fine, delicate connective tissue, well supplied with bloodvessels. This adipose element forms cushions, which act as protection to underlying structures. It is found more especially in the soles of the feet and palms of the hands, mammary gland, especially after child birth, also about the external sexual organs, back and shoulders. Besides the blood-vessels found in this layer, we also have the coils of the sweat glands, also some of the deeper seated hair follicles.

The bloodvessels consist of two systems, the deep in the subcutaneous tissue and the superficial immediately beneath the papilla; they are said to be more numerous in the flexor than in the extensor surface of extremities.

The papilla of the hair has its own arteriole which branches into looped capillaries. Nerves are both of a medullated and non-medullated variety, which richly supply the skin, usually derived from the subcutaneous branches accompanying the bloodvessels. They generally terminate between the epithelium and the rete mucosum.

The medullated nerve-fibres end in those strange bodies, known as Meissner's corpuscles, commonly known as tactile corpuscles. These tactile corpuscles are little rounded bodies usually situated in the papilla or beneath it; they are quite numerous in the finger tips. They are from $1/250$ to $1/300$ of an inch long to $1/500$ broad, different varieties being found in the different parts of the body.

Sudoriferous glands are small globular shaped bodies, yellowish in color, embedded in the subcutaneous connective tissue and opening with a small duct on the surface of the epidermis. They are smaller on the eyelids, nose, and largest around the areola of the nipple, the base of the scrotum and axilla. Sometimes they attain the size of one-tenth of an inch. The duct generally emerges between the papillæ. They make their appearance in the fifth month of embryonic life. They have a good nerve and blood supply and are found in great numbers all over

2

the body; 2,685 are found in a square inch. The length of one uncoiled tube is about one-fourth of an inch. The sum total of Krause's numeration in an adult would exceed nine miles of perspiratory function, which gives us some conception of the importance of this wonderful eliminating process of the much neglected, though nevertheless wonderful, organ of the skin. The secretion of these glands depends somewhat on the location of the gland, which, of course, modifies the secretion, but it is usually a clear, watery fluid.

Sebaceous glands, or, as they are sometimes called, glands of the hair follicle situated in the corium, found from the outer root—sheath of the hair. They are divided into three groups: First, those of the scalp, beard, and axilla, or in the region where hairs are coarse and fully developed; second, those connected with the lanugo; third group is where the glands open directly upon the skin and are not connected in any way with the hair follicle, as are found in the external surface of the prepuce behind the corona glandis in the male, and in the female on the surface of the nipple, the vestibule, and the labia majora. They vary in size in different parts of the body, are largest on the eyelids (the meibomian), mons-veneris, labia majora, scrotum and anus. They are whitish in color, consisting of an external basement membrane and an internal epithelial lining, and usually open into a hair follicle. The secretion is largely a fatty matter.

The Hairs—Hairs are modified epithelial tissue, cylindrical, slender in structure, and embedded in the depression of the skin, known as the hair follicle. Each hair is divided into two portions, the root embedded in the skin and the shaft which projects above the skin. They are found all over the body except on palms of the hands and soles of the feet, last phalanges of fingers and toes. Hairs are divided into three classes, long hairs, as of the scalp, beard, and axilla; second, those of the eyebrows and eyelids, and third, fine, soft lanugo covering other parts of the body.

The cortical portion of the hair is composed of flat fusiform epithelial scales. The centre or medullary portion consists of embryonic corpuscles, which are quite often pigmentated, that gives shade or color to the hair; it is closely connected with the amount of pigmentation in the skin. Gray and blonde hair has very little pigment. The hair follicle in which the root is imbedded is a pouch-like connective tissue structure consisting of three layers, the external, middle and internal. It consists of connective tissue containing an artery. vein and nerve.

Nails—Are also modifications of the epidermis, differing from it by being harder and firmer. They are horny, elastic, translucent plates, embodded in the skin and attached to the dorsum of the phalanges. They have four borders, the anterior being free, the posterior and lateral, slightly curved longitudinally in their natural state, convex on their upper surface, but in latent syphilitic patients they are spoon shaped, and flattened, very thin, having lost their natural curve.

Nails are supposed to be a modified portion of the Stratum Lucidum, beginning its function in the third month of intra-urine life, and by the eighth month a greater part has developed.

PHYSIOLOGY OF THE SKIN

An organ like the skin, of such complex and wonderful structure, could not possess a less wonderful and complex function; usually the work of the internal organs is confined to one or two functions, but in the skin we find its functions are more varied and more numerous than that of any other organ in the body; therefore, a study of its function is of even greater importance to the physician than its anatomy, who especially should be familiar with those internal disturbances of the life force that so frequently present themselves upon the external surface of the body or the skin. Like the barometer, it shows the rise and fall of the mighty disturbing forces within. This may be well illustrated in acute exanthematous diseases. How quickly do we see the circulatory storm subside, the gastric or catarrhal symptoms grow less, as soon as the eruption is fully developed upon the skin. None the less true is this in many of the deep chronic disturbances, but whose relationship is not so clearly shown to the untrained observer.

Of the many offices of the skin, five special ones might be mentioned. First, it protects the deeper tissues and organs beneath. As a garment it is folded and tucked about us, protecting us from mechanical irritation, the action of the atmosphere and irritating substances; second, as a sense organ; third, for the regulation of the temperature; fourth, as an organ of secretion and excretion including perspiration; fifth, absorption. The fatty cushions in the connective tissues, besides the elasticity and firmness of the corium, modify the effects of blows and other mechanical injuries that might otherwise affect the internal organs or tissues beneath. The nature and structure of the horny layer of the epidermis prevents the too rapid transudation and evaporation of the fluids of the tissues; otherwise, the evaporation of the water of the fluids of the body would be continuous, and to such an excess that the tissues would dry up and death be the result.

It further protects against irritating substances, also high and low temperature; however, the regulation of the body's temperature is one of the most important offices of the skin, maintaining it at a fixed standard. The increase or decrease of a few degrees below or above normal being incompatible with life, but owing to the power of resistance the skin is endowed with, it is able to resist even greater variations each day.

The skin being a very imperfect conductor of heat, it, therefore, protects the body against heat and cold by the retention within the tissues of a considerable portion of the heat. It is said to have a separate apparatus for heat, cold and pressure, therefore, in an irritation of the skin, the sensation does not depend so much on the kind of irritation as upon the property of the nerve endings.

The principal means of sustaining the normal standard of temperature is by the process of cutaneous transpiration; by the impression of warm or hot air on the vaso-motor nerves of the skin, the cutaneous muscles become relaxed, the bloodvessels dilated and general superfices of the skin increased. The skin becomes suddenly bathed with perspiration, and by means of rapid evaporation active heat is changed or converted into latent heat and the temperature of the perspiring surface rapidly diminished. This is more marked in humid air than in dry, enabling one to endure a very high temperature in a dry air, where he would not be able to endure such a temperature in a corresponding moist atmosphere. As long as the perspiration is not interfered with, a great degree of heat can be endured.

The sebaceous and sudoriferous glands perform the secretory and excretory functions of the skin. The sebum or sebaceous matter is a semi-fluid, oily matter, consisting of palmitin, olin, saponified fats, and other fats of the blood. Its principal purpose is its action as a lubricator, keeping the skin moist and pliable, and preventing a too rapid evaporation from cutaneous surfaces, also protecting the skin against dampness or excessive moisture and external infection.

The secretion of the sweat glands is a colorless fluid of a slightly salty taste, although it may be alkaline or acid in its reaction, under certain pathological conditions. It is 99½% water, with certain organic acids and a number of salts of the blood. It is quite volatile, easily evaporating. There are two forms of perspiration, the sensible and the insensible. The quantity excreted daily varies greatly in different persons, of course influenced very much by their employment, but the average is from one and a half to two pounds. It is controlled by the central nervous system, existing probably in the spinal cord and medulla.

Absorption, the last function mentioned, by means of which a great number of substances of a gaseous or medicinal nature are absorbed or carried into the circulation, more especially by means of wearing apparel and by the never-to-be-thought-of noxious custom of local medication upon the surface of the skin, such as mercury, quinine, camphor, turpentine, arsenic, and other substances.

SYMPTOMATOLOGY

The symptomatology of the skin is usually classified as in other diseases into objective and subjective, or symptoms referring to structural changes or alterations in the skin recognized by sight or touch, while the latter classification is referred to those disorders of sensation cognizable only to the patient.

The symptomatology is by no means confined to the skin itself, but may involve any part or organ of the body. The true homœopath recognizes all diseases, whether upon the skin or not, as first a disturbance of the life force or the internal dynamis, and that the symptoms that manifest themselves upon the skin are simply a reflection or external expression of the internal change; and that the internal economy is usually relieved by such an expression. For pathological purposes, the objective or external signs upon the skin are frequently sufficient, but for a higher therapeutic purpose a fuller comprehension of the true relationship between the pathological and the primary internal disturbances must be known, in order to be able to cure our cases by the administration of the internal homœopathic remedy. In our anatomy and physiology of the skin, especially its minute anatomy, we saw the numerous offices it had to fill, frequently taking place at times to a very great degree of auxiliary organs, such as the kidneys, and having imbedded within itself such a complex system of secretory apparatus, besides being richly supplied with lymphatics, nerves and bloodvessels; hence, the apparent possibility of each part becoming the seat of morbid action or change.

"Pathological conditions of the skin are further magnified by the strong sympathetic relationship existing between the nervous system and the skin, it being the receiver of all sensory changes from without and from within, by its vaso-motor and trophic innervation, it becomes the principal medium through which are reflected disorders of the central nervous system from toxemias and from functional and organic disturbances of the viscera."

Lesions—The lesions of the skin which have been classified into primary and secondary, may develop singly or multiple in each individual case; even very different pathological conditions may have similar lesions. Frequently a diagnosis can be made at once by a study of the lesions that present themselves, and again it may require a succession of changes before we are assured of the nature of the disturbance.

PRIMARY LESIONS	SECONDARY LESIONS
Macules	Excoriations
Papules	Ulcerations
Pustules	Fissures
Tubercles	Crusts
Vesicles	Cicatrices
Bullæ	Squamæ
Wheals	Pigmentation
Tumors	

Macules—Synonyms: Maculæ or spots.

Macules include all varieties of circumscribed discolorations of the skin. They are usually round or oval, but vary in size and shape, from a pin-head up to several square inches, and their color may be any tint or shade, depending on the diseased conditions. They are on a level with the skin and may or may not disappear under pressure. They are classified into erythema, purpura, and vascular spots.

Papules—Synonyms: Papulæ; pimples.

Papules are small, solid elevations of the skin of new formation; size from a pin-head to a split pea. They may be of the normal color, and are either round, flat or conical, even umbilicated. Papules are usually caused by an inflammatory process, and their duration is variable. They generally disappear by absorption, but may be converted into pustules.

Pustules—Synonym: Pustulæ.

A pustule is simply a vesicle with purulent contents.

It may originate as a pustule or may develop as a papule or vesicle, although the change from one lesion to the other may be so rapid that the form is not recognized. They are superficial or deep, the former leave no scar, but the latter by the greater destruction of tissue leave a permanent scar. The nature of their contents gives color to the pustule; therefore, they may be any color from yellow to red, even purple. They terminate by rupture or dessication, sometimes leaving crusts behind, as in eczema, herpes or impetigo. They are quite often surrounded by an inflammatory areola.

Tubercles—Synonyms: Tuberculæ; nodules.

Tubercles are solid circumscribed formations from the size of a pea to a hazelnut. The distinction between tubercles and papules is frequently one of size; the latter is, of course, more superficial, while the former consists of a deeper cellular infiltration into the corium. The evolution is much slower than the papule; their borders definitely defined, and their tops flat. They may be of the normal color of the skin, although their color varies with the nature of the inflammatory process.

Vesicles.—Synonym: Vesiculæ.

Vesicles are small, round or oval elevations of the skin, from the size of a pin-head to a split pea, usually of an inflammatory origin and formed by an exudation of serum or sero-purulent liquid under the skin; their color varies according to their contents; a typical one is transparent and contains pure serum. They may be superficial or deep, depending on the nature of the lesion. They are of short duration, disappearing by absorption; sometimes, however, they coalesce in patches or group themselves together, as in zoster; successive crops are not uncommon.

Bullæ—Synonym: Blebs.

Bullæ may be regarded as large vesicles of round or oval form and of almost any size, containing a serous, sero-purulent, or bloody fluid, the color depending on the nature of its contents and the time of its retention. It may be straw colored, bloody, or even black.

Wheals—Synonyms: Urticæ; pomphi.

Wheals are circumscribed inflammatory lesions of the skin of various sizes and shapes, due to an œdematous infiltration into the papillary layer of the corium, usually with a pink areola. They appear or disappear very suddenly, leaving no trace of any lesion behind.

Tumors—Are large, solid elevations of the skin, of all sizes, generally spherical in form, usually flesh colored, but may be of various hues, due to disease changes. They are frequently due to new growths or to changes in sebaceous glands or from retention of sebum.

SECONDARY LESIONS

Excoriations—Synonym: Abrasion.

Excoriations are losses of substance from the superficial layer of the skin due to traumatism. They may be of any form or shape, generally torn points, or linear shaped wounds, similar to those found in scratch marks or from sharp pointed instruments. They may be deep enough to form crusts over them.

Ulcerations—Synonym: Ulcers.

Ulcerations are inflammatory breaches of continuity, due to suppuration and destruction of the superficial tissues. This loss is usually replaced by cicatricial tissue; they may be of any size or depth, their edges sharp-cut and well defined, everted or undermined; their bases may be smooth, but are generally uneven and filled with broken down tissue or bathed in pus or serum. Crusting is not uncommon and healing takes place by the formation of a cicatrix.

Rhagades—Synonyms: Cracks, fissures.

Rhagades are linear lesions involving the epidermis and upper layers of the corium. They are usually produced by muscular contraction, when the skin is dry, hardened and thickened, due to inflammatory changes. They are almost always found in the palms of the hands and soles of the feet, phalanges of fingers and toes, and flexure of the joints; occasionally we find them upon the lips. Patients suffering from this lesion are usually tubercular.

Crustæ—Synonyms: Crusts; scabs.

Crusts are concretions of matter due to the dying up of secretions. They vary in color, depending on the nature of the exudation; they may be any form or size. When removed they usually leave an ulceration or cicatrization. They are greasy and yellow in seborrhœa, sulphur-colored and cupshaped in favos, greyish black or green in rupia.

Cicatrices—Synonym: Scar.

A scar is a new fibrous tissue growth, due to the replacing of lost tissue by ulceration or other process. It is covered by an epithelial layer; glands, hair follicles, papillæ are absent; nerves and bloodvessels are not numerous. Two forms are recognized, the atrophic and hypertrophic. They are of a pale pink color at first, but become white and often glistening with age. If superficial, they are soft and movable; but if deep seated, they are hard, uneven, and immovable. Their form and size depend on the nature of the lesion. They are of great diagnostic value.

Pigmentation—Pigmentation is an augmentation in color, usually of a circumscribed portion of the skin, due to many conditions; congestions, inflammations, trophic changes, formation of neoplasms, diseased conditions of the organism; as in diseases of the liver and spleen, syphilis, or as found during gestation.

SPECIAL LESIONS

When the lesions are gathered into groups or separate areas or fields of diseased surface, it is said to be in patches; these patches, taken as a whole, constitute the general eruption. These patches may be represented in the form of circles, ellipses, etc.; again they may follow certain lines, as the direction of a nerve distribution, as seen in herpes zoster.

Lesions are spoken of as punctuate, when occurring in points or small dots; nummular, when size of a small coin; miliary, when the size of a millet seed; lenticular, of the size of a pea or bean; acuminate, when they are pointed; plane, when they are flat; umbilicated, when they are depressed on their centers.

When lesions are separate they are said to be discrete; when they run together, confluent.

Patches.—When arranged in circles or segments of circles, are said to be circinate; when in rings, annulate. The patch is serpiginous when the lesion is advancing from one edge and healing at the opposite edge; when limited in its extent, it is said to be circumscribed, but when spread over a large surface, diffuse.

ETIOLOGY

Probably no organ of the body is diseased from so many various causes as that of the skin; being so intimately associated with all the internal organs, it must naturally become sympathetically affected by any disturbances in the organs themselves, be it hepatic, gastric, intestinal or pelvic. From whatever source it may originate, the skin must in some way assist in the eliminative process, or receive reflexly in some degree the force of the organismic disturbance; again, while we may study the many disturbing influences from within, whether of a toxic nature or not, we must remember that a world of toxic influence comes from without; hence, the necessity of an etiological division. Two divisions or classes are recognized by all writers; they are the symptomatic and idiopathic, those which involve more or less the organism, and, secondly, those causes which act directly upon the skin.

The practitioners of Hahnemannian Homœopathy look upon the predisposing cause of disease from a far different light than all other therapeutists or students of pathology. Well they know that all diseases or disturbances of the life force have their primary origin in one of the chronic miasms, psora, syphilis, or sycosis. That all the eruptive diseases can be traced directly or indirectly to one or more of these, and in this work we shall from time to time call your attention to these underlying or basic miasms in each disease.

Thus under predisposing causes we may embrace all conditions pointing to a miasmatic origin, such as eruptive fevers, nutritive disturbances, hereditary conditions, well advanced miasmatic states, such as debility, anemia, plethora, and diathesis.

Eruptive Fevers.—Many of which affect the whole organism, and as a marked feature of their presence the skin is often seriously involved. Some of the severe types are found in scarlet fever, rotheln, measles, chicken-pox,

2

vaccinia, and small-pox. The history of these diseases points, first to a specific involvement of the organism by an infectious agent, to be immediately followed by a secondary involvement of the skin, so that each infectious agent produces, secondarily, a specific lesion which seems to be a part of an eliminative process of the infective agent.

Nutritive Disturbances.—The skin is frequently involved by changes in the nutrition of the body, thus in a rheumatic or gouty diathesis we may have hemorrhages into the skin, eczema, certain forms of herpes, moles, warts, psoriasis, boils, carbuncles, erysipelas, even gangrene.

Hereditary Conditions.—In hereditary conditions we find that very psoric patients are subject to innumerable diseases of the skin, such as eczema, acne, etc. Deep and far-reaching are the influences of heredity, explainable only to those who have made a careful study of the miasmatic origin of disease. Conditions known as general debility, anemia, plethora, faulty nutrition are but the outgrowth of psora, syphilis, or sycosis in a latent state, that has been slowly undermining, probably for years, the vital forces of the patient; frequently brought to the surface by the well selected antimiasmatic remedy, and the whole organism is relieved of its suffering as if by magic.

Age, Sex, Climate.—May in a sense be classified as predisposing causes, which have much to do in influencing those miasmatic changes in the different cycles or turning points of life, as in infancy, puberty, and at the climacteric changes. Few of the malignancies occur until the age of forty is reached.

Effect of climate has a marked and often a very serious influence upon patients suffering from some deep-seated chronic miasm, especially in extremes of temperature as in tropic zones, and as seen in such diseases as leprosy and other malignancies; again diseases that run a mild course in some latitudes may develop alarming constitutional symptoms in others.

SECONDARY CAUSES

Among the secondary causes we may enumerate errors in diet, drugs, vaccination, improper clothing, heat, cold, medicinal and chemical irritation, personal habits, parasites.

Drugs.—Among the drugs a few may be mentioned that have a marked action upon the skin, which, taken as a whole, may produce almost any lesion known in diseased states, such as *antipyrin, copaiba, turpentine, quinine, chloral, belladonna*, the *bromides, iodides, cantharis, chloroform*, certain acids and chemicals. These are to be studied separately, as they simulate often disease lesions and disease conditions.

Dietetic Errors.—Dietetic errors induce a great number of cutaneous diseases, especially in those patients who are predisposed to suffer from certain kinds of food. They seem to lack the power to assimilate them to any degree, frequently inducing such diseases as pruritus, urticaria, erythema acuta, etc. Among those which produce the above-named lesions most frequently are fish, oysters, shell fish, strawberries, oatmeal, buckwheat, cheese, rich foods, especially when lard is used in the making of pastry.

Vaccination.—Vaccination may be considered both an exciting and predisposing cause, as the system has no power within itself to eliminate the effects of this deep chronic poisoning; therefore, through hereditary transmission, it becomes predisposing cause as it becomes co-existent with the life force.

The frequency with which the majority of human beings are being inoculated with this specific poison, as it is only a specific poison that will produce such a malignant pustule as is seen in vaccination, firmly implants on each organism a constitutional basis fruitful to the production of numerous diseases of the skin as well as any other organ of the body.

Chemical Irritation.—The chemical irritants that may come in contact with the skin in innumerable ways are the effects of the sun's rays producing dermatitis and often pigmentation and various other lesions, strong soaps, poisonous plants, such as the nettle, rhus tox, sumac, etc. The majority of the rhus family produce in sensitive subjects erythema, vesicular eruptions and even true inflammations of the skin.

Mosquitoes, bees, insect bites of all kinds, strong alkalies or acids.

Mechanical Irritation.—The mechanical irritation varies with the habits and the employment of man; the excoriations, bruises and lacerations are the result of mechanical causes; men who work much in water develop eczema. Bakers develop from the irritating influence of the flour the disease known as baker's itch. Masons, plasterers, workers in oils, and leather workers develop diseases peculiar to themselves.

Personal Habits.—Personal habits offer a fruitful field for investigation, as frequently many of the existing causes can be traced to the habits of the patient; eczema and acne rosacea are commonly the results of alcoholic indulgences, over-eating, excessive smoking and especially the cigarette habit, or personal uncleanliness in general.

Improper Clothing—Clothing has often much to do in producing various forms of pruritus, eczema and other forms of diseases of the skin; more especially is this true in the use of flannel underwear, colored hose, dyed with impure or irritating materials. Smooth and finely woven linen or cotton materials produce less irritation of the skin and are to be prescribed to the preference of all others made from silk or woolen.

Parasites—Many of the most annoying diseases of the skin are due to animal and vegetable parasites, such as are seen in the different forms of tinea, scabies, etc., affecting not only the skin but the hairy scalp and nails.

Pathology—The more important pathological changes of the skin for our consideration are anemia, erythema, hyperemia, inflammation, hemorrhages, hypertrophy, atrophy, the formation of new growths and parasites. Any or all layers of the skin may become involved, but the corium is usually the principal one affected, probably due to its great nerve and vascular supply. It is frequently the seat of attack from numerous animal and vegetable parasites, neurotic disturbances, disorders of the sudoriferous and sebaceous glands or their ducts.

Anemia—Anemia is due to a deficient amount of capillary blood; it may result as a loss of blood or an impoverishment due to diseased conditions of the general system. It is characterized by unnatural pallor, and it may take on a cachectic, greyish or yellowish tinge, and as a rule a decrease of the surface temperature and sometimes diminished sensibility. Circumscribed anemia may be produced by cold, local anaesthesia or injuries.

Hyperemia—Hyperemia is due to an increased amount of blood to the vessels of the corium; it may be active or passive. The active may be produced by internal causes, or from heat or cold, or from the application of local irritants. It is recognized by a bright red color of the affected part, which disappears by firm pressure, only to return as soon as it is removed. Such sensations as tingling or burn-

3

ing, heat, etc., may be present; even the temperature of the part may be elevated.

The active form is generally of brief duration, and the skin resumes its normal appearance. Pigmentation may occur and sometimes becomes permanent, even desquamation may take place.

Hyperemia sometimes passes into true inflammation.

Inflammation—Inflammations of the skin are the same as inflammations elsewhere, as far as the phenomena are concerned. In the beginning is a stage of active congestion followed by infiltration and exudation, even to a complete stasis of the circulation and destruction of the part. Other lesions may present themselves, which complicate the case, such as vesicles, papules, pustules. The inflammation usually involves the corium and subcutaneous connective tissue at first, and later on invades the epidermis; it may terminate by absorption or go on to suppuration.

Hemorrhages—Hemorrhages are usually caused by a rupture of the capillaries of the corium. The amount of blood extravasated depends on the plasticity of the bloodvessels and the severity of the primary cause. It may occur in simple lines, as in vibices, or in little dots, as in petechia, or in large patches, as in ecchymosis.

Hypertrophy—Hypertrophies are abnormal enlargements in normal tissue, either of pre-existing elements, or new elements. It may be limited to one or more layers of the skin. In clavus, corns and warts both the epidermis and corium are involved, but in elephantiasis all the layers are affected.

Atrophy—Atrophy is a decrease in either the size or number of the elements of a tissue. It is due to a trophic disturbance of the system and may be circumscribed or general.

New Growths—New growths are neoplasms, whose structures differ from the original tissue, as seen in cicatrix, keloid, fibroma, etc. It is a new histological development into the substance of organized structure. The lymphatic bloodvessels and nerves may be involved, and a new growth partake of one or more of these specified tissues.

Parasites—A parasite is an animal or vegetable organism that draws its existence or living at the expense of another. They are the source of a large and annoying family of skin diseases. They are not satisfied with the invasion of the skin itself but attack the hair, hair follicles, and even the nails. Many of these parasites, especially the vegetable, are microscopic, of which the trichophyton is typical.

DIAGNOSIS

To be a successful diagnostician of diseases of the skin, the physician must cultivate, above all other faculties, his powers of observation and touch, as the majority of the cases we meet must be diagnosed principally from these two sources of help. Of course, a carefully taken personal and family history will be of valuable assistance to us. A glass of considerable magnifying power is almost necessary in order to study the nature of the lesion intelligently; even the microscope may be required to distinguish, more especially, between specific or non-specific, malignant or non-malignant conditions. But among the necessary conditions to be remembered are light, temperature, sex, age, and social conditions. Every case should be examined under good light, and above all others sunlight. The best time for examination is in the morning or forenoon. The temperature of the room should be 68 or 70 degrees, as it is a well-known fact the skin becomes mottled on exposure to cold, in sensitive patients. In exanthematous diseases the eruptions recede and become often quite indistinct. Age and sex are to be considered for reasons already mentioned, social conditions and vocation are not to be neglected, besides regional distribution of the lesions, color, odor, primary and secondary lesions, subjective symptoms, such as itching or the absence of it, the absence or presence of constitutional symptoms, besides the general evolution of the lesions.

CLASSIFICATION

The factors taken into consideration in the classification of the diseases of the skin are their pathogenesis and their clinical similarity. They are also classified from a pathological, etiological, and anatomical basis. They are governed by the same pathological laws governing morbid processes in other organs of the body.

Of course having such an imperfect knowledge of their causes prevents us from making any true etiological classification, therefore, any system may be looked upon as being provisional and subject to such modifications as the progress of our knowledge demands.

Classifications—1st. Erythemas; 2nd. Inflammations; 3rd. Hemorrhages; 4th. Hypertrophies; 5th. Atrophies; 6th. New growths; 7th. Neurosis; 8th. Diseases of excretion and secretion; 9th. Parasites.

PART II

CLASS I—INFLAMMATIONS

THE EXANTHEMATA

Scarlatina—Synonym: Scarlet Fever.

Scarlatina—Is an acute self-limited, contagious, febrile disease, characterized by a diffuse scarlet rash over the whole or greater part of the body, and accompanied by a severe inflammation of the throat; and although it may run a mild course, constitutional symptoms are generally severe. It is divided into four separate stages. First, Period of incubation; second, Prodromal; third, The stage of eruption; fourth, The stage of desquamation or decline.

Symptomatology—It generally begins with a chill or chilliness, headache, nausea, vomiting and sore throat, following a period of incubation, lasting from five to six days.

The fever rises rapidly, with a temperature of 102 to 104. The skin is dry and intensely hot, tongue furred, great dryness of the throat, face flushed, pulse quite rapid, often in children from 140 to 150. The eruption makes its appearance on the second day upon the face, neck and upper part of the chest; within twenty-four hours it covers the entire surface of the body. It is usually more intense around the flexures of the joints; sometimes small pin-head vesicles appear on the surface during the development of the rash, the throat symptoms increase in severity, the tongue becomes red and papillated. (Characteristic strawberry tongue) The fever remains at its height until the fifth or sixth day, when it begins to decline; this, of course, is greatly influenced by the treatment. The throat symptoms lessen and the constitutional symptoms gradually disappear, the eruption disappearing in the order it first made its appearance. This is followed by desquamation of the epidermic layer of the skin, to a greater or less degree, sometimes desquamating in large flakes.

The above symptoms are characteristic of the simple form of scarlatina. However, sometimes the disease manifests itself in severer forms, which are known as *irregular forms*. They are also known as scarlatina maligna, hæmorrhagic and anginosa.

Malignant Scarlatina—This is also known as the ataxic form. A child in apparent good health becomes suddenly ill, complaining of a severe pain in the head, vomiting, the countenance cyanosed, pulse rapid, and the patient soon lapses into an unconscious state, with more or less violent delirium, followed by coma and death. In these cases the temperature often rises to 105 or 106, and the patient is overwhelmed by the intensity of the poison, often even before the eruption makes its appearance.

HÆMORRHAGIC FORM—Extravasation of the blood takes place under the skin and mucous membrane, accompanied frequently by hæmorrhages from the bowels or internal organs; these usually begin at the appearance of eruption. These cases are usually accompanied with great prostration, but there may be active delirium accompanied by convulsion, coma, and followed by death in two or three days.

THE ANGINOSE FORM—In this form the throat symptoms develop with alarming intensity, resulting in great swelling of the fauces and tonsils, together with the formation of diphtheritic or false membrane, which although easily detached is apt to extend to the larynx. Ulceration and even gangrene of the larynx may follow, accompanied by great fetor of the breath. The glands of the neck become very much enlarged, and a severe inflammation of the connective tissues generally.

COMPLICATIONS—The diphtheritic inflammations of the throat, or larynx, or abscesses; heart complications, such as pericarditis, endocarditis or otitis media, resulting from the extension of the inflammation from the pharynx by the way of the Eustachian tube. In tubercular patients, meningitis, even albuminuria, is a common sequel at the close of the desquamative stage, which may develop into a chronic condition known as scarlatina brightii. The other probable complications are pulmonary edema, pleurisy, bronchitis, and broncho-pneumonia.

MORBID ANATOMY—In a study of the morbid anatomy of the skin, we find the cells of the rete swollen and the bloodvessels distended; ecchymosis may be found beneath the serous and mucous membrane. The lymphatic glands of the neck are usually much swollen as well as the tonsils; the mucous membrane of the pharynx intensely congested and sometimes ulcerated, and in the malignant forms congestion of internal organs is frequently met with.

Etiology—All cases arise from a specific virus, either directly or indirectly. The contagion may be conveyed from one patient to another, or indirectly through letters, books, clothing, etc. Contagion may be carried long distances. Ninety per cent. of the cases are to be found in children, although no age is entirely free from it, all depending upon the susceptibility of the patient. As a rule, one attack immunes a patient from further attacks. It is said to be more contagious during the disquamative stage.

Diagnosis—The principal diagnostic points are the suddenness and violence of the symptoms in the invasive stage, sudden rise of temperature, and the rapid pulse, with pain and soreness of the throat, followed by the characteristic eruption.

Prognosis—The prognosis varies in different epidemics, depending on the different forms that the disease assumes. It is more severe in the tubercular and strumous patient, and especially severe in adult life. A temperature of 105 and over is indicative of a severe form of the disease. Nephritis is also a serious complication.

Treatment—Probably no disease has brought forth greater laurels to the homeopathic practitioner than his treatment of scarlet fever, both as to the efficacy of the remedies, which has reduced the time and sufferings of these patients fully fifty per cent.; besides, the development and direction of the disease action proves fully and positively the law Hahnemann laid down in his organon, that all eruptions should make their appearance from within outward, and from above downward, and disappear in a similar manner. If you will examine the throat and hard palate of these patients, you will find the first appearance of the eruption in that region, whether it be of this disease or measles, showing that from the great centers of life by which the organism is governed in health, it is also governed in disease, therefore the course of the eruption, which is the physical expression of the internal disturbance, is in the direction of the action of the normal life force; hence the cure ought to take place the same way.

The treatment should follow the principles as laid down in all febrile diseases. The patient should be put to bed and kept there until convalescence takes place, and the diet should consist of milk and such liquid nourishment as all fever patients should have, special attention being given to the secretion of urine, always watching for albumen, for with such a severe and extensive inflammation of the skin, its eliminating process is greatly impaired and the work thrown almost entirely upon the auxiliary organs, the kidneys. Much bathing is objectionable in all diseases of the skin, so great care is to be exercised in bathing such a large diseased surface, for fear of chilling the body and producing stasis; that, with the objectionable method of rubbing much fatty matter or oils upon the skin, has much to do with a stasis to other parts. The intense pruritus following the desquamation can always be removed speedily by the well-selected homeopathic remedy. The remedies most frequently employed in simple forms of scarlatina are Aco., Bell., Bry:, Rhus tox., Puls., Apis., Ars., Gels., Lyc.

MALIGNANT FORMS—Ars., Apis., Arum triph., Ailanth., Carbol. ac., Kali b., Lach., Nitr. ac, Phyto., Pyrogen., Carbo veg., Lac can., Mer. bin., Mer. prot. iod., Phos., Lyc.

Aconite—Full, quick pulse, dry, hot, burning skin, much mental and physical restlessness, thirst for large drinks of cold water, quick, rapid breathing, peevishness and revolt against all interferences.

Belladonna—Belladonna is probably more frequently indicated in the simple forms than all other remedies, as its pathogenesis more frequently meets the pathogenesis of each case. Face flushed, patient usually drowsy, apathetic, takes frequent naps, the eruption very smooth and red, marked strawberry tongue, full bounding pulse, throbbing of the carotids, thirst for frequent sips of water, frequent fits of delirium, with startlings in the sleep, throat very sore, dry, red, with no saliva, frequent empty swallowing, skin dry, hot, burning to touch.

Bryonia.—Usually small pulse, severe frontal or general headache, desire to lie quiet and aggravated by motion generally, thirst for large drinks of cold water, tongue dry, white coated, often bitter taste, usually tight, dry, hard cough which aggravates the headache, face pale, desire to be left alone, irritable, cross, subject to pleuritic and rheumatic pains.

Baptisia—Headache, backache, very weak, drowsy, stupid, confused mentally, tongue brown, dry, face dusky and has a besotted look, low forms of fever of a typhoid nature.

Rhus tox—Much aching and soreness in the muscles, bed feels hard, great physical restlessness, with desire to change position often, which gives temporary relief, cannot lie still in any position, worse from cold, better by heat and by motion, muscles sore and stiff, eruption takes on a dusky hue, often vesicular.

Gelsemium—Low forms of fever, patient drowsy, sleepy, great muscular weakness, trembling of the hands, basilar headache, cerebral intoxication, pulse frequent, soft, weak, eyes heavy looking and suffused, muttering delirium when asleep or half awake, twitching of the muscles.

Arsenicum—Typhoid forms with delayed eruption (Bry.), great prostration, mental anxiety and great restlessness, mouth and lips dry, great thirst for frequent sips of cold water that often produces vomiting, great debility, anxious, restless, fear of death, irritable, sensitive, peevish, worse after one o'clock at night or in the afternoon, skin dry, burning, itching, better by heat and by lying with the head high.

Pulsatilla—(Sang-lymp-temp.) With blue eyes, light

hair, pale face, indecisive, slow, weeps easily, affectionate, mild, gentle, timid women. Symptoms constantly changing, chilly, yet worse by heat and when the room is warm, thirstless, mild forms of scarlet fever.

Malignant Scarlatina—(Remedies) *Lachesis*—Advanced or malignant cases, tongue dry, dark red, trembling, inability to protrude it, patched or mapped, throat dark bluish color, neck sensitive to touch, throat worse on the left side, extremely painful swallowing, pain extending to the left ear, dark, offensive looking membrane, tendency to paralysis of the throat during convalescence, sensation of restriction about the throat, fears they will choke to death, all the symptoms worse after sleep.

Lac Caninum—Symptoms similar to Lach. generally worse on left side, but disposition to change suddenly from side to side is characteristic of the soreness, ulcers and pain. Pain worse one day on the left, next day on the right. Sore throat almost disappears then returns again. Ulcers or diphtheritic deposit usually very dark, sometimes shiny, or has a glazed appearance. Sensations as if the throat was closing and she would choke; this seemed between the throat and nose (Lach. around the throat). This remedy is as frequently indicated in sore throat as the mercurius, and acts best in a single dose of the high potency.

Lycopodium—(Sang-ment-temp). Very severe cases of sore throat, beginning on the right side, diphtheritic deposit brownish red, spreads from right to left, worse from cold drinks, worse after four o'clock; child drowsy, sleepy, wakes from a sleep frightened, seems to know no one; soon they drop to sleep again only to awaken with the same symptoms. The deep blood poisoning shows itself by the marked diphtheritic symptoms extending often to the posterior nares and even infiltration of the lungs, much tympanitis, urine scanty, dark red, albuminous.

Apis—Much chilliness, no thirst, great edema of throat. Uvula looks like a sac of water, stinging pains in the throat on swallowing, tongue and mouth dry, inability to swallow; urine scanty, high colored, oppressed respiration, in the delirium the patient is inclined to scream out, puffed condition of the hands and face, abundance of albumen in the urine. Tendency to anasarca with post scarlatina conditions, and to brain complications, stinging, biting in the skin, much restlessness and nervous agitation.

Arun triph.; Malignant Forms—Stopping up of the nose and posterior nares with membranous deposit, discharge from the nose excoriating upper lip and nose. Ulcers in the mouth and throat, saliva acrid, tongue red, papillæ elevated, putrid sore throat, swollen submaxillary glands.

Ailanthus—Adynamic form, marked prostration, cerebral disturbances, livid eruption, skin dry, hot, vomiting often with muttering delirium. Photophobia. Dry, parched tongue, with great thirst, throat congested with glandular swelling, mental torpor, great exhaustion, petechiæ. Eruptions irregular, patchy, slow to appear, interspersed with small vesicles.

Pyrogen—Pyrogen is indicated where there are marked septic conditions with a tendency to decomposition of the fluids of the body, septic ulcers, abscesses, etc. There is great restlessness, with a constant desire to move, like Rhus tox. patient moans and complains constantly, frequent rigors with extreme coldness, often with persistent vomiting, followed by severe aching of the bones and extremities, breath horribly offensive, all discharges offensive, tongue clean, smooth, dry, fiery red, cracked, brown or black, thirst for cold water which produces vomiting.

For pulmonary complications. Remedies to be thought of are Bry., Phos., Ars., Kali phos., Lyc., Hepar, Amo., Carb., Tub. Otitis and otorrhœa: Mer. viv., Lyc., Psor., Puls., Cal. c., Nat. mur., Sil., Hepar, Teuc., Tub.

Anasarca—Apis, Ars., Mer., Sol., Berb., Vul., Phos., Blatt. orient.

MEASLES (MORBILLA)

DEFINITION—Measles is an acute contagious, eruptive, febrile disease characterized by the development upon the skin of a papular eruption over the entire body and accompanied with a catarrhal inflammation and irritation of the mucous membrane of the respiratory passages. It is very contagious to children, but not exclusive to them. There are two forms, the simple and malignant.

SYMPTOMS—The stage of incubation lasts from ten to twelve days, but may be even of a shorter or longer period. It may commence with a chill or even with general malaise, followed with muscular soreness, headache, and to all appearances with general symptoms of a cold. The coryza is thin and watery, frequent sneezing, eyes congested, suffused, conjunctiva red with dread of light. The symptoms are accompanied by an eruption, rise of temperature, dry irritating laryngeal or bronchial cough. The voice is harsh and husky, more or less congestion and redness of the throat. This period lasts from three to five days, followed by a lentil-sized papular eruption beginning on the forehead and face, and frequently spreading over the body from above downward, completing its course in about three days. The color of the rash is deep red or purplish. Pruritus is often present; about the third day after the appearance of the rash; the fever, cough and catarrhal symptoms gradually begin to disappear the sixth day; the bronchial cough may continue for some time. Desquamation begins about the sixth day, proceeding rapidly over the body. The scales are much smaller than those of scarlet fever. Occasionally a mild form of diarrhœa is present, but usually the bowels are constipated.

Malignant Measles—This form is of very rare occurrence, but when it does occur it presents symptoms of a typhoid nature, represented in pulmonary complications or in hæmorrhages with extravasation of blood beneath the mucous and serous membranes, or from the various orifices of the body. A secondary attack of measles seldom occurs.

Complications—Inflammation of the larynx, bronchitis, lobar pneumonia, otitis media, conjunctivitis, whooping cough occasionally accompanies it, and convulsions sometimes occur in very young children.

Etiology—All children seem to be predisposed to measles, at least they seem to have less immunity than from any other of the diseases of children, unless it be whooping cough. The age most susceptible seems to be from three to five years. It is extremely contagious and frequent epidemics occur from exposure in schools, waiting rooms, and public gatherings. It may be conveyed from the breath, exhalations from the skin, or from any of the secretions of the body, from clothing, books, letters, etc. It is contagious at all periods. March and April are the prevailing months for epidemics in this latitude.

Diagnosis—Diagnosis is somewhat similar to common coryza or la-grippe in its earlier symptoms, but the presence of an epidemic; the prolongation of the fever; the peculiar eye symptoms; the eruption with its peculiar shot-like feeling, are quite diagnostic.

Prognosis—The prognosis is quite favorable.

Pathology—The pathology shows that hyperemia of the capillary vessels of the cutaneous papillæ, followed by slight exudation into the surrounding tissue, and congestion of the respiratory mucous membrane.

Treatment—Rest in bed and warmth promote the progress of the eruption. Great care should be taken against chilling the body until the desquamative stage is fully passed, as it endangers complications.

REMEDIES—*Aconite*—In the beginning, where there is dry, hot skin, rapid, full pulse, red, watery eyes, photophobia and general anxiousness and restlessness of aconite, dry, hacking cough.

Belladonna—Frequently follows Aconite, presenting a similar circulatory phenomena, hard, full, bounding pulse; drowsiness, sleepiness, marked congestion of the eyes, dilated pupils, dry intensely hot skin, dry, tight, short, irritating cough, giving no rest, face flushed, eruption quite red, twitching of the muscles with a tendency to convulsions in children. Thirst for frequent drinks of cold water.

Bryonia—The eruption is slow in coming forth, bilious motive temperament, dry, tight, painful cough, frontal headache, very irritable, constipation, nausea on sitting up, thirst at long intervals for large quantities of cold water, tendency to chest complications.

Rhus tox—General soreness of the muscles, great restlessness and desire to change position, lameness and stiffness of the muscles, restlessness, in the after part of the night, aggravated by uncovering: dry short, teasing cough, caused by tickling under the sternum, dark red measly rash accompanied with intolerable itching, followed by an inclination to become vesicular.

Gelsemium—Much chilliness, much lachrymation, and profuse watery discharge from the nose, hoarseness, soreness and rawness in the chest, prostration of the whole muscular system, headache in the cervical spine, general drowsiness and sleepiness, eruption a livid color.

Pulsatilla—Negative patients of a mild, yielding disposition who complain of chilliness, yet who are made worse by heat, mild forms of fever with dryness of the mouth, yet without thirst, aggravation in the afternoon and in the evening, better in a cold room, from eating or drinking cold things. Loose cough with expectoration of thick, yellow mucus, inflammation of the eyes with marked yellowish discharge. Tendency to weep.

Arsenicum.—Great anxiety with much mental restlessness before the rash makes its appearance, constant craving for cold water, drinks little at a time, vomiting and loss of strength, all the symptoms worse after midnight, persistent burning heat of the skin, dry mouth and lips.

Remedies for further consideration are Ant. crud., Carb. veg., Coff., Dros., Euph., Hep., Lach., Mer., Phos., Spong., Sulph., Ham., Dolic., Cham., Nux vom.

RUBEOLA

SYNONYMS: Roseola; rotheln; German measles.

Rubeola—Is another of the exanthematous diseases of children, partaking partially, it would seem, of the nature of morbilla and partially of the nature of scarlet fever, yet still independent of either. There are four reasons given why it should be considered a distinct affection from either of these diseases. 1st. Its epidemic qualities. 2nd. Its incubation, invasion and eruptions differ. 3rd. It attacks indifferently and with equal intensity subjects who have had both of these diseases. 4th. It attacks only those who are exposed to the special contagion.

Symptomatology—It appears in epidemics usually in the winter or spring. The stage of incubation is from ten to fifteen days, yet there is no positively stated time. The prodrome is short, the eruption usually making its appearance during the night; in fact, the breaking forth of the eruption is among the first symptoms of the disease. It appears first upon the face and spreads rapidly all over the body. Its color is pale red, which disappears on pressure, a slight pruritus accompanies it, and on a close examination of the rash we find it is composed of small lentil-sized papules, diffuse, irregularly disseminated and frequently grouped as in measles. Sometimes it resembles measles, and again more distinctly scarlet fever; the eruption lasts from one to three days, disappearing entirely or nearly so, then reappearing. The catarrhal symptoms are usually in proportion to the fever, although the coryza is often absent, the bronchial cough is rare; there is more or less redness, dryness and soreness of the throat, and swallowing is sometimes quite painful; the temperature seldom rises above 102. Complications are rare, yet bronchitis, pleurisy, pneumonia, and albuminuria are reported in a few cases.

Diagnosis—The principal points are the mild course of the disease, the slight catarrhal symptoms, the enlargement of the cervical glands and the history of the patient having had measles, and the absence of the dry, tight, rasping cough of measles. In scarlet fever the constitutional and throat symptoms are more severe, the rash is finer, more diffuse and less papular in its nature.

4

Etiology—It is a disease of childhood, and occurs usually from the age of five to fifteen, generally among the poorer classes.

Prognosis—Prognosis good, complications rare.

Treatment—The same as in measles and scarlet fever.

VARIOLA (SMALL-POX)

DEFINITION—Variola is an acute, specific, contagious febrile disease, marked by the presence of an eruption upon the skin, which is at first macular, then papular, vesicular, and finally pustular, followed by crusting. It is accompanied usually by severe constitutional symptoms which are most prominent during the stage of invasion and suppuration. Clinically speaking, there are four classes or forms. Discrete, confluent, varioloid, and hæmorrhagic or purpuric (black small-pox).

Symptomatology—The disease is ushered in by a chill, or a succession of chills, less severe than the first (after 10 or 12 days of incubative period, more or less). This is followed by a temperature ranging from 101 to 104 and accompanied with severe backache in the lower lumbar and dorsal region; aching in the lower extremities, frontal headache, loss of appetite and sometimes nausea and vomiting, tongue dry, coated, red at the sides, eyes suffused, face swollen; in severe cases there may be marked delirium, and epistaxis is common in children.

The skin is usually dry, but there may be profuse sweating. At this stage of the disease the so-called *initial rash* may appear, of which there are two varieties, the diffuse or scarlatinal, and the macular or measly, either of which may be accompanied with *petechiæ*.

The rash may be general, or limited to the abdominal region or the extensor surface of the body; these rashes are usually purpuric in their nature, or partake of an erythematous blush; they occur in from ten to fifteen per cent. of the cases and usually about the second day. The eruption usually appears on the forehead on the fourth day in a discrete form, in small red spots; within twenty-four hours it appears in other parts of the body; as the rash subsides, the temperature and general symptoms modify and the patient feels better. About the fifth day the papular eruption changes into a vesicular one, each being elevated, circular and slightly umbilicated; about the eighth day they become pustular, flat and assume a globular form, and of a greyish or yellowish color, with quite a marked injection of the areola. The temperature again rises and a secondary fever returns lasting from twenty-four to forty-eight hours in the discrete form; about the tenth or twelfth day the fever departs and convalescence begins; on the fourteenth day desquamation is far advanced; very little pitting takes place in this form; of course it all depends upon the severity of the case. The amber colored crusts often remain imbedded in the skin for sometime, but finally fall off, leaving the peculiar scarring or pitting known in this disease.

Variola Confluent—This variety has the same clinical symptoms except they are greatly intensified in each stage. The chill, headache, backache, fever, eruption, all are greatly magnified, the mucous membrane of the mouth and throat is much swollen and edematous, covered with pustules, the parotid and sublingual glands are swollen. Erysipelas is a frequent complication. The temperature often rises to 105 or 106; the disease assuming a low typhoid form, convalescence is, of course, much protracted with more or less sloughing and destruction of the tissues.

Variola Maligna—The symptoms of this form take on

a specific and malignant nature from the beginning, a severe and prolonged chill ushers in the disease, temperature frequently is 107, vomiting, collapse, comatose conditions follow in rapid succession, the urine is often suppressed, dysenteric stools, exreme backache and pain in the limbs accompanied with scarlatiniform or erythematous eruptions, papules blue and even black with hæmorrhagic extravasation which are prone to coalesce, tongue thick, black, showing hæmorrhages into the mucous membrane, urine dark, bloody, albuminous, and often before the appearance of the eruption the whole body becomes discolored.

COMPLICATIONS—Complications are remarkably few considering the nature and severity of the disease. Laryngitis, bronchial pneumonia, (endo- or myo-carditis rare).

Prognosis—A low death rate in the simple form but quite unfavorable in the hæmorrhagic form.

Diagnosis—No mistake ought to be made in this disease as soon as the eruption appears, as it is so unique and distinct from all others; yet some difficulty may be met with in the beginning due to the initial scarlatina or measly rash, but these do not occur frequently.

Treatment—Remedies—Acon., Apis, Ars., Bapt., Bell., Bry., Camph., Carbol., Carbo veg., Carbol. ac., Coff., Cundur., Hyos., Kali bi., Gels., Mer. Sol., Phos., Phos. ac., Rhus tox., Sarracen. purp., Sulph., Medorrh., Syph., Tart. emet., Tart. crud., Thuja, Variola, Verat. vir., Lach., Lyc., Lac can., Mur. ac., Nat. mur., Nit. ac., Nat. sulph., Pet., Psor., Puls., Pyrog., Rhus rad., Sanic., Sep., Sil., Tub., Zinc., Varicell., Crotal., Crot. tig., Anac.

It is a well known fact that during the epidemics of small-pox the total mortality from all diseases, including small-pox, is lower than during other years.

The treatment is both prophylactic as well as general.

As to the use of prophylactics in this disease it is sometimes necessary, but do not overstep the law of similia; do as you would in other contagious diseases, such as scarlet fever, measles, diphtheria, etc.

The patient and all those who have come under the contagion should be isolated, which is the best method to prevent the spread of the disease. Pasteur saved the silk worm industry of France some years ago, when they were suffering from a plague that would seem as though it would annihilate every silk worm in France, by speedily removing the diseased worms from among the healthy. Careful and scientific nursing, which means in addition plenty of fresh air, cleanliness, and a suitable diet, will do much towards assisting the physician in curing these patients. As to the question of vaccination we have no space to discuss the matter, either pro or con. We simply condemn it as a prophylaxis, as we do all forms of sero-therapy. Our motto is, "Prophylaxis through health and not through the propagation of disease." The virus of commerce is simply human variola conveyed to the animal, and therefore it is a serum product, made by a similar process to that which all other serums are made and used by sero-therapeutists, which is, of course, a degenerative process, and when we call into account those serums, such as are used in diphtheria, tuberculosis, hydrophobia, and tetanus, being only used in diseased persons, their danger cannot be compared with that of vaccinia, which is in such universal use to-day as a prophylactic, since compulsory vaccination forces it upon the healthy, as well as upon the unhealthy of all ages, even to the infant in its mother's arms.

The potentized virus has been proven sufficiently by

those who have used it to be far more effective as a prophylaxis, and does not carry with it a septic poison.

REMEDIES—*Aconite* is sometimes indicated in the first stage of the disease, especially where there is great restlessness, much erethism and great fearfulness, and apprehension of an unfavorable termination of the case. Suitable to full-blooded bilious or sanguine bilious temperament, hot, dry skin with great thirst and nervous tossing about.

Ammonium mur—Hæmorrhagic diathesis, stout, fleshy people who have a tendency to hæmorrhages, putrid sores in the mouth and throat, or cholera-like symptoms, developing during the course of the disease, especially where the eruption does not make its appearance in the lower portions of the body.

Apis mel—May be useful in the earlier stages where there are erysipelatous swelling with stinging pains, great soreness of throat, and absence of thirst, scanty dark-colored urine. It is indicated in irritable, nervous, fidgety people, who are hard to please. Puffiness of the hands and feet with a tendency to anasarca; better in a cool room, and by bathing with cold water.

Arnica—Poorly developed eruption with ecchymosed spots, here and there accompanied with a sore, lame, bruised feeling throughout the body, as if beaten; complains of great heat of the head and of hardness of the bed; low forms of fever.

Arsenic—Malignant or hæmorrhagic forms of smallpox, irregularly developed eruption, with typhoid tendency; the pustules are filled with a dark-colored fluid; great exhaustion and sinking of the vital forces; anxiety and fear of death; great thirst, but water often produces vomiting; aggravation in the afternoon or after midnight; much burning in the lesions.

Baptisia—Sanguine or Bilious Motive. Typhoid symptoms; fetid breath; sordes on the teeth; pustules in the nasal cavity. Great prostration, with decomposition of fluids (Pyr.); ulceration of mucous surfaces; all discharges and excretions very offensive; tongue dry, yellowish brown center, later on cracked and ulcerated; mentally confused, imagines the parts of his body are separated; much nervousness; face dusky; drowsy; tendency to hæmorrhages.

Bryonia—Severe splitting headache; thirst with desire for large quantities of cold water; great nausea, faintness and even vertigo on rising from a recumbent position; dry, parched lips; the patient lies perfectly still, because motion aggravates all the symptoms; eruption very indistinct.

Carbo veg—Asthenic variola, with cold breath and coldness of points remote from the center of circulation; excessive prostration; great desire for fresh air and to be fanned. Eruption livid, purplish, breath and all excretions of the body have a carrion-like odor.

Hamamelis—Hæmorrhagic small-pox with dark passive venous hæmorrhages, oozing of dark blood from any of the different orifices of the body. Venous, congestion, low passive typhoid states.

Lachesis—Malignant small-pox, extreme cases, eruptions dark, coalesce, malignant looking, very sensitive to touch, great physical and mental exhaustion, malignant pustules, dark bluish, or purplish in appearance, much stupor and muttering delirium as soon as he falls asleep; tongue dry, dark, trembles on protruding it; discharges thin, dark, offensive; all the symptoms worse after he falls asleep.

Mercurius sol—Very apt to be indicated in a pustular

stage; discharges bloody; all the symptoms worse during the night; tongue large, thick, flabby, showing the imprint of the teeth; much offensive tenacious saliva in the mouth; marked tendency to formation of ulcers on mucous surfaces; metallic taste or complete loss of taste; eruptions bleed easily; profuse perspiration; much thirst; slimy, bloody, dysenteric stools; trembling of the hands; aggravation from warmth.

Phosphorus—Is especially adapted to tall and slender persons where there is a tendency to lung complications, hemoptysis, burning of the hands and feet, great weakness, with nervous debility and trembling, longs for cold food, icecream; heaviness and weight on the chest, larynx sore, raw, painful; worse lying on the left side; pustules filled with blood.

Phosphoric ac.—Vesicular looking pustules; patient is dul and stupid, cares for nothing, notices nothing, wants nothing; delirium, muttering, unintelligible; lies in a stupor or stupid sleep; apathetic, in low febrile states.

Rhus tox—The disease assumes a typhoid type from the beginning, excessive restlessness, constantly tossing about, no rest in any position; sordes on the teeth and lips; tongue dry, cracked; confluent small-pox, eruption livid, bloody pustules; much aching and soreness of the muscles; better by heat and by change of position.

Tartar emet—The rash is slow in making its appearance; the disease assumes a typhoid putrid type, much nausea and vomiting; thick, white, pasty coated tongue; face cold, blue, pale, covered with cold sweat; rattling of mucus in the bronchi; tendency to paralysis of the lungs.

Variolinum—Proving imperfect, although it has done splendid work in the treatment of the disease, much used as a prophylaxis; the higher potencies are to be perferred.

Remedies for further consideration: Puls., Ant. cr., Canth., Chin., Secale, Sil., Stram., Sulph., Ipec., Hyos., Hepar, Hyd., Cham., Camph., Melan., Thuja.

VARICELLA (CHICKEN POX)

Definition—An acute contagious eruptive disease, affecting principally children, marked by the development of a vesicular eruption on the surface of the body; seldom seen after the tenth year.

Symptomatology—Stage of incubation ten or twelve days, usually begins with a slight chill, followed by febrile symptoms, though often the fever is unnoticed and the eruption shows the first appearance of the disease; the eruption consists of small vesicles or bullæ quite superficial, somewhat grouped; they contain a clear serum, and are surrounded by a reddish halo. The eruptions disappear in about a week leaving no scar or mark. The disease is quite severe sometimes in adults.

Etiology—Rarely found in children after ten years of age, more frequently met with from the third to the seventh year; one attack generally produces immunity. It is less contagious than variola, not so easily conveyed by clothing, and is said to be produced by inoculation with difficulty. It may exist sporadically or in epidemics.

Diagnosis—The mild prodromal symptoms, the sudden appearance of the vesicular eruption in successive crops.

Prognosis—Very favorable; no fatal cases reported.

Treatment—Preserve the warmth of the body, cleanliness and regulate the diet. The remedies to be most frequently consulted are Bry., Puls., Rhus tox., Bell., Acon., Gels., Mer. sol., Vario., Ant c.

ERYTHEMA

DEFINITION—Non-contagious superficial hyperemia of the cutaneous surface. It is characterized by redness and swelling of the skin. It usually appears in patches non-elevated, disappears on pressure, leaving a yellowish tinge which immediately reassumes its red appearance. It generally disappears by a desquamation, and is usually accompanied with more or less heat, tingling or burning. There are two forms, the simplex and the idiopathic, but by most authors this has been divided into many subdivisions, such as erythema neonatorum, traumaticum, caloricum, intertrigo, besides the symptomatic forms, which are: Erythema roseola, infantilis, erythema medicamentosum, erythema scarlatiniform, erythema bullosum and nodosum. The line of division between hyperemia and true inflammation of the skin is not a positive one; the distinction is often made simply for clinical convenience. In erythema the symptoms are entirely local, while in true inflammation the symptoms cannot always be confined to the local surface.

SYMPTOMATOLOGY—The symptoms differ according to the form of the affection which may be present; the redness may be diffuse or concrete, in children it is often punctuate. All degrees of redness are met with, from a pink to a deep or dark livid red, and it may become bluish, even cyanotic where there is marked venous congestion. It may or may not be painful. The symptoms, of course, vary according to the form.

PATHOLOGY—The simple form is generally due to dilatation induced by a disturbance of the vaso-motor nerves. Either it generally depends on local causes, reflex or some internal intoxication.

Erythema Neonatorum—This disease manifests itself

in new born children, and is characterized by a general diffuse redness accompanied with local elevation of the temperature. It first appears as a pale flush, and gradually deepens to rosy red, but in four or five days it gradually disappears by desquamation. Sometimes it assumes a marked icteric hue, due probably to the changes in the liver that take place at that time. It is occasionally accompanied with quite a marked pruritus.

Erythema Traumaticum—It is a diffuse redness of the skin confined to the injured part; if the disease is of a severe nature other lesions may appear, such as eczema, bullæ, pustules, vesicles, ulceration, or even gangrene. It results from mechanical irritation coming in contact with irritating substances, prolonged wetting of the part, secretions, pressure from tight clothing, etc.

Erythema Caloricum—This form of erythema is induced either by cold, heat, or exposure to the sun's rays. It is diffuse and limited to the part exposed; it may become chronic, and show a marked pigmentation, which is slow to disappear.

Erythema Intertrigo—The simple form of erythema is usually due to the friction of two surfaces lying in apposition to each other, or it may be due to prolonged moisture, irritating discharges, etc. The locations of the disease are usually in the inguinal regions, flexures and folds of the body, especially where there is much adipose tissue. It begins with a diffuse redness, followed by a thin or purulent exudation.

The discharges are usually offensive, and the lesion may go on to crusting.

Roseola Infantilis—This form is due to or has its origin in gastric derangement, dentition, or intestinal irritation, or arises during the course of inflammations of internal organs. The eruption consists either of macules or a punctate rash distributed over the body; it remains but a short period, gradually disappearing without desquamation.

Erythema Medicamentosum—This form is produced by the action of irritating drugs, and will be dealt with more fully later on in this work.

Erythema Scarlatiniform—This is a non-contagious, symptomatic eruption characterized by a diffuse red rash, resembling scarlatina, due to some reflex vaso-motor disturbance.

SYMPTOMS—The constitutional symptoms vary with the cause. There may or may not be any febrile symptoms, but it usually begins with a general *malaise*. There is generally more or less chilliness, with a marked rise of temperature, followed by a sudden appearance of the rash. The temperature does not always subside, however, at the appearance of the rash. The rash may appear suddenly after the invasion of the prodromal symptoms, or it may be two or three days before it makes its appearance. It usully extends all over the body, except the face, which is apt to be free from it; it proceeds rapidly, may be diffuse or punctiform and of a bright scarlet red color; occasionally minute vesicles are present; there is usually much burning, prickling and itching. It disappears in from one to five days with more or less desquamation, especially about the articular surfaces. A few cases are mentioned where the entire epidermis of the hand was thrown off. The tongue is usually coated, red at the sides and tip. There is a marked tendency to relapses in the disease.

Pathology—The pathology is quite obscure.

Etiology—It appears to be due to reflex vaso-motor

disturbance; following wounds, disease conditions, or from the ingestion of certain kinds of foods, such as shell fish, fruit, vegetables, or from the administration of anesthetics, alcoholic poisoning, from drugs, such as Opium, Quinine, Mercury, Belladonna, Copaiba, Antipyrine, etc.

Diagnosis—It is distinguished from scarlet fever by the absence of the marked throat symptoms, and strawberry tongue, and the early desquamation, also the absence of complications.

Prognosis—Prognosis is usually good, much depending upon the primary cause; of course if the cause is due to any profound disturbance of the system emanating from such diseases as pyemia, septicemia; or puerperal conditions, it would make the prognosis decidedly unfavorable.

Erythema Bullosum—Bullæ may be either a primary or a secondary affection. They may be located separately upon the skin or there may be a secondary lesion on a primary erythematous base. Their contents are usually at first transparent, but it soon becomes turbid, sometimes purulent, and even bloody, and during the drying up process sometimes thin yellowish crusts form over them. It may be accompanied with severe itching and burning.

The lesions occasionally develop on the nose, lips, tongue and buccal cavity. Some of the gravest forms of erythema are bullous in their character.

Erythema Nodosum—This form is usually ushered in by chills, fever, rheumatic pains, gastric disturbances. The eruption is usually located on the tibiæ or on the arms; it may, however, occur in other parts of the body. They present themselves in roundish oval-shaped nodosities, generally grouped, vary in size from a hazelnut to that of an egg. They are at first bright red, painful to touch, generally accompanied by a dull, aching and burning sensation. They gradually become darker, assuming in their formative course almost any shade or color They do not ulcerate.

The disease is subject to relapses or to appear annually. The duration of the eruption is from three to six weeks.

Etiology—Erythema nodosum occurs more frequently in younger people, especially in women. It develops in tubercular patients, debilitated or poorly nourished subjects, sometimes with a complication of rheumatism or malarial symptoms. Kali iodide is said to have produced this lesion.

Pathology—It seems to be idiopathic in its origin, morbid anatomy. It is an exudation due to inflammatory process through all the layers of the skin.

Diagnosis—The location of the disease, the arrangement and the changes in color in its development which is from a dusky red to blue, green even black.

Prognosis—Prognosis good. Relapses occur until the constitutional dyscrasia is removed.

Treatment—Neonatorum — Remedies — Aco., Arn., Ars., Apis, Cham., Lyc., Puls., Sep., Sulph., Nux v., Rhus t., Urtica urens.

Lycopodium—Lycopodium is one of the most frequently indicated remedies in this disease. Skin yellowish red or red with a marked icterous hue; much flatulence and belching of gas, constant rumbling and rolling in the bowels; bowels tympanitic; much drowsiness when free from pain, and screams for hours when suffering from flatulence. Urine scanty, dark, containing a reddish or yellowish sediment with an aggravation of all the symptoms at four o'clock.

Aconite—The infant is feverish, hot, restless, sleepless, and is in much distress.

Belladonna—Skin very red, dry, hot, shiny, hot to the touch, pulse rapid, full, hard; fever makes the child drowsy.

Bryonia—Constipation, large, dry, stools; much thirst; vomits after nursing; desires to keep perfectly still; better lying on right side.

Cal. carb—Child perspires profusely about head and face when asleep, so as to wet the pillow. The child is irritable, wilful; skin very yellow with general calcarea symptoms.

Chamomilla—Indicated in very sycotic children; discharges from the bowels greenish, sour, acrid, excoriated; child very irritable, screams as if angry; warm sweat about the head; desire to be carried about.

China—Much tenderness in the region of the liver, profuse sweating all over the body as soon as it falls asleep; digestion very weak, vomiting or diarrhœa as soon as the child nurses or partakes of food; diarrhœa profuse, yellowish water, followed by a limp prostrated condition of the whole body.

Mercurius sol—Tenderness and soreness in the liver, all the symptoms are worse at night; much salivation, swelling of the glands, slimy or bloody stools with tenesmus.

Nux vom—Constipation, stubborn, frequent urging, and ineffectual; child is worse after nursing, cross, irritable, better by heat in general; skin very yellow.

Hepar—Tendency of pustules to form, which are filled with a bright yellow pus, intertrigo following excoriations from urine or other discharges; any abrasion of the skin heals slowly and is very sensitive to touch; always much suppuration, cervical glands large and tender to touch.

Sulphur—Dry, pimply, unhealthy skin, skin full of papules with much itching, discharges from the body excoriate, symptoms worse by heat.

Erythema Traumaticum—The remedies for consideration are Arn., Bell., Bry., Rhus tox., Bel. per., Sulph. ac., Staph., Ledum, Hep.

Erythema Caloricum—Belladonna. The part is dry, hot, smooth, shiny, sensitive to touch, may or may not be any temperature.

Rhus tox—The erythema takes on a bluish appearance, with a tendency to vesicate, vesicles containing a straw-colored serum or a bloody pus, much burning and itching, which is worse on exposure to the air.

Cantharis—Bullous forms with marked vesicle irritation.

Petroleum—Much heat and burning in the part; chronic conditions after frost bites, painful itchings, chilblains, worse in the winter, better in the summer; moist eruptions, covered with pustules with copious purulent secretion, or dry, cracked and bleeding easily.

Agaricus—Indicated in people with light, lax muscular fibre, poor circulation, sensation of the skin as if ice touching it, or of hot needles piercing the skin; chilblains itch and burn intolerably, or extreme redness of the part with intolerable itching and burning; parts red, swollen, hot, extremely sensitive to cold.

Erythema Intertrigo—Remedies: Acon., Ars., Borax, Graph., Hep., Lyc., Mer. sol., Rhus, Cal. c., Petrol., Sulph., Syph,, Tub., Medo., Psor., Caul., Led.

INDICATIONS—*Arsenicum*—Great burning and itching, thin, watery, excoriating discharges. The discharge produces an erythema on parts passed over; symptoms ameliorated by heat.

Borax—Dark erysipelatous-like inflammation in groins, folds and flexures of the body of young infants with a tendency to form pustules on inflamed surfaces, often accompanied with a dread of falling, or of a downward motion and other symptoms of Borax.

Graphites—Strongly indicated in tubercular or latent syphilitic patients with dry, easily cracked, thin, sensitive skin; erythema of a dark bluish color, either dry, cracked or bleeding, or secreting a sticky, honey-like secretion, worse in fall and spring or in snowy weather.

Hepar—Secretions very copious, yellowish and often offensive; part very sensitive to touch, better from warm bathing; slightest abrasion of the skin suppurates; very sensitive to cold and desire to cover up warmly.

Sulphur—Dark red, dry, rough, pimply eruption, accompanied with much itching, which is worse by warmth of bed, worse by bathing; great burning and smarting after scratching; deep chronic psoric conditions.

Psorinum—Pale, delicate, sickly children who have poor reaction, and who are very sensitive to cold, skin unhealthy, dirty looking; hair dry, lustreless; erythema dry, scaly or moist, oozing a sticky, offensive fluid, better by warmth and perspiring.

Tuberculinum—Adapted to light complected patients with a family history of tubercular affections; chilly patients who take cold easily, knowing not how nor where; morose, irritable, fretful, peevish children; discharges greenish yellow; itching worse when undressing.

Medorrhinum—This remedy is indicated in the diseases of children where there is a parental history of sycosis. Discharges and secretions excoriate and produce a bluish erythematous eruption, or the discharges produce intense

5

pruritus. Often this sycotic condition is recognized by red moles or spider spots upon the skin, warty formations, gouty conditions or gouty concretions; colicky pains and sour smelling stools.

Reseola Infantilis—In this form of erythema, being of symptomatic origin, no special set of remedies can be enumerated for study as the causes are so numerous and varied. However, those remedies acting more directly on the gastro-intestinal tracts are to be given careful consideration.

Erythema Scarlatiniform—For the treatment of this form of erythema we will find some assistance in following closely the indications given under the treatment of scarlet fever and measles.

Erythema Bullosum—Remedies for consideration are: Ars., Apis., Canth., Rhus tox., Nat. mur., Dul., Lach., Mer. sol., Nit ac., Caust., Gum. gut., Juglans cin. For indications see under Pemphigus.

Erythema Nodosum—Remedies: Apis., Arn., Bry., Con., Lach., Nux, Rhus tox., Sulph. ac., Cal. c. China, Dul., Puls., Sil., Sulph., Ledum. See indications in simple erythema.

ERYSIPELAS

Synonyms: Rose or St. Anthony's fire.

Erysipelas is an acute, specific, eruptive, febrile disease, slightly contagious, usually endemic in its character, but sometimes epidemic; prevalent more particularly in the spring of the year.

It is characterized by intense localized inflammation involving the skin, mucous membrane, and the superficial lymph vessels. There are two forms, idiopathic and traumatic. We, however, recognize these as one and the same thing, as the traumatism is only an exciting cause. The phlegmonous forms will not be treated here as they are not a true erysipelas.

SYMPTOMS—It usually begins with a chill, although there are many cases that have no perceptible cold stage. Temperature usually rises from 101 to 104, accompanied with such constitutional phenomena as follows any marked febrile condition.

LOCAL SYMPTOMS—Within twenty-four hours the eruption makes its appearance; on examination we find a dark red, edematous, swollen, irregular and slightly elevated patch, which spreads more or less rapidly, depending much upon the intensity of the inflammatory process. On pressing the fingers over the lesion a yellowish color appears, but it immediately resumes its red, livid appearance. The amount of swelling depends much on the locality of the disease; if upon the head or face where it most frequently makes its appearance, there being a great amount of loose cellular tissue, we frequently find the parts enormously swollen and disfigured. The eyelids are frequently so enormously swollen as to prevent the lids from being opened for days. Soon the parts become tense, shiny, red and indurated; owing to the excessive exudation into the epidermis, sometimes vesicles or even bullæ form upon the surface; occasionally these become pustular and form crusts. Even a gangrenous condition may follow, due to pressure and closure of the lymph channels. The erysipelas remains stationary for a number of days; but when under proper treatment quickly recedes, and ends by the constitutional symptoms gradually subsiding, and the lesions disappear by desquamation.

Pathology—Erysipelas is said to be an inflammation of the skin due to the streptococci as described by Fehleisen;

but to-day we know that the above-named streptococcus is identical with the streptococcus of suppuration. The disease is, no doubt, of sycotic origin or sycosis implanted upon a well-marked psoric base. And like all other severe acute diseases, it manifests itself in a more malignant type on those patients with a tubercular diathesis.

MORBID ANATOMY—A sero-fibrinous exudation and infiltration of small, round cells. The connective tissue fibres of the corium are swollen and the lymph spaces are dilated.

Etiology—The primary cause, as has already been attributed to the streptococci of Fehleisen, which we do not agree with; however, such local disturbances as surgical operations and other wounds, parturition, vaccination, etc. often readily assist in the development of the disease, and yet we have idiopathic cases developing with probably greater frequency, where there is no lesion to assist in the development of the streptococci. The simple fact of the matter is the true cause of disease exists within the individual himself, and all external exciting causes simply assist in the developing or propagation of that internal and ever present condition.

Diagnosis—The disease may sometimes be mistaken for acute eczema, but the constitutional symptoms are usually absent. Except in young children, similar constitutional symptoms may arise, but they are only temporary. If proper attention is given to the clinical symptoms in the early course of the disease, together with the progress, extension and character of the lesion, the diagnosis is easy.

Treatment—The local treatment is cleanliness of the part and occlusion of the air, which lessens or modifies the local symptoms.

REMEDIES—*Aconite* in the early stage, and especially

in children; where there is quick, rapid pulse, hot, dry skin, much delirium, restlessness and throwing themselves about the bed, indicated previous to the appearance of the eruption.

Belladonna—High fever, full bounding pulse, throbbing of the carotids, flushed face, sleepy, drowsy condition of the patient; lesion very red, smooth, shiny; skin intensely hot.

Rhus tox—Indicated in rheumatic patients where there is much aching in the back and limbs; great physical restlessness, with impatient desire to change position frequently; lesion dark red with a tendency to vesicate.

Anthracin—Erysipelas-gangrenosa with typhoid symptoms; great pain in the head and dizziness; delirium and unconsciousness, great depression and prostration; copious perspiration; sleepy, drowsy stupor.

Apis—Great edema of the part; skin often pale, doughy-like to touch, or bullous forms; sac-like swellings filled with transparent serum; burning, stinging, prickling pains; parts very sensitive to touch; tendency of disease to go from right to left; scanty high-colored urine. > in the cool air.

Arnica—Phlegmonous erysipelas with extreme tenderness and soreness to pressure. Bullous forms; the part is hot, hard, shiny, swollen, deep red; the patient has a sore, bruised feeling all over, or the bed is too hard; erysipelas following bruises or contusions.

Lachesis—Lachesis is indicated when it begins on the left side of the face or body rapidly spreading to the right; the lesion is dark blue, very sensitive to touch, cannot bear the weight of clothing or even dressings to touch it; a tendency to a phlegmonous condition; patient is generally worse after sleep.

Lac caninum—Lac caninum is indicated in nervous, restless, highly sensitive organisms. Symptoms very erratic. Both local and constitutional symptoms are constantly changing, now better in one way, now worse in another, and vice versa. The disease begins with an intense, unbearable backache. The lesion is dark blue, the patient is despondent, hopeless, irritable, fears to be alone.

Ledum—Ledum is indicated in very gouty patients or from erysipelas following the bites of insects. It usually begins on the left side and follows a mild chronic course; worse at night and worse by warmth.

Lycopodium—Lycopodium is for right-sided erysipelas, where the disease spreads from right to left. Typhoid forms.

Remedies for further study are: Canth., Bry., Euphorb., Puls., Borax, Graph., Rhus rad., Tereb., Mer., Phos., Carb. veg., Sabin., Plumb., Vinca m., Stram

FURUNCULUS (FURUNCLE, BOIL)

DEFINITION—It is an acute circumscribed inflammation of the hair follicle and surrounding connective tissue, ending in abscesses.

SYMPTOMATOLOGY—The lesion begins in a small pinhead, red papule, accompanied with a slight itching and burning. Within forty-eight hours the area of redness becomes more extended and infiltration more marked. In the course of a few days the lesion becomes fully formed and appears in a round or conical tumor with a small pustule on its apex. Pain is of a throbbing character, intensified by contact or motion; generally worse at night. In a few days later it breaks open, discharging a greenish, yellowish or bloody pus; and finally a dead piece of tissue, known as the *core*, is thrown off. When the local symptoms subside it heals rapidly. There are two forms, the follicular and the cellular. They invade any region of the body, but by preference the neck, face, axilla, back, buttocks, genital regions and extremities. They are frequent complications of eczema, scabies or prairie itch.

Diagnosis—The diagnosis is easy. It differs from carbuncle from being smaller and having only one point of suppuration.

Pathology—Due to some derangement and obstruction of circulation.

Etiology—It usually occurs from some constitutional derangement or impairment of the nervous function, or from inactivity of any of the internal organs, due to overeating, local irritation or pressure.

Treatment—Rectify hygienic conditions, removing all possible dietetic causes, such as coffee, pork, salt meat, cheese, pastry, shell fish.

REMEDIES—Nux, Bry., Puls., Hep., Lyc., Mer. c., Mer. sol., Nat. c., Nitr. ac., Nat. mur., Sulph., Sil., Iod, Cal. c., Chin., Graph., Fluor. ac., Rumex, Nux jug., Tub., Psor., Medor.

CARBUNCULUS (CARBUNCLE)

DEFINITION—The carbuncle is a circumscribed, deep-seated inflammation of the skin and subcutaneous tissue, terminating in a slough. In the beginning it is sometimes difficult to distinguish it from a common boil; but as a rule, it starts out with symptoms of a more serious character. It is usually ushered in by a chill followed by fever. The part becomes hot, dusky red, circumscribed. The area affected is often from one to three inches in diameter. The pain is of a dull or throbbing character. Later on the skin becomes of a dark bluish red, tense and shining. But by the end of a week or ten days the whole mass begins to soften, and the skin breaks at two or three different points. Pus and a necrotic-core is discharged from each opening. The swelling, tension, due to the infiltration of plastic lymph., recedes, and the cavity gradually fills in by granulation. The size, flatness and the numerous points of suppuration, together with the gravity of the constitutional symptoms, distinguishes it from furuncles.

The favorite sites are back, neck, shoulder, buttock.

Pathology—The inflammatory process begins in a hair follicle. The area of the necrotic patch is in direct proportion to the resistance the skin presents in different parts of the body.

Prognosis—Favorable where there is no deep-seated disease, such as in diabetes, alcoholics, or in old people.

Treatment—Heat in the different forms is soothing and often quite beneficial in the early inflammatory stage, but such surgical interference as curetting or lancing is not advisable. Care, however, should be taken to keep the part surgically clean, as the numerous suppurating points offer favorable means for absorption and infection.

REMEDIES—Anthrac., Ars., Apis., Bell., Bry., Bufo, Carbo veg., Carbol. ac., Chin., Lach., Nitr. ac., Puls., Rhus tox., Sep., Sil., Pyro., Taran., Cub., Mur. ac., Nux, Mag. phos., Tub.

INDICATIONS—*Anthracin.* Violent, burning pains. Erysipelatous inflammation, hæmorrhagic infiltration, cerebral symptoms, glandular swellings, and a general gangrenous destruction.

Arsenicum—Indicated in pale anæmic patients where there is great prostration, much restlessness and fear of death; burning pains, or the part burns like fire; discharges thin, often bloody; acrid and excoriating; much thirst; pain and local symptoms better by heat.

Lachesis—Carbuncle dark, bluish red color, extremely sensitive to touch; discharge dark, thin, ichorous pus, very fetid, bleeds easily. The carbuncle is often surrounded by purple spots; symptoms worse after sleep.

Apis—Great swelling and edema of the part, stinging pains; better by moistening the part with cold water; no thirst.

Carbo veg—Where the disease takes on a very malignant type, and the discharges are dark colored, foul smelling and very offensive. Carbuncles on old people where there is much prostration, the tendency to gangrene accompanied with a carrion-like odor.

Tarantula—Adapted to highly sensitive, nervous organisms. Carbuncle dark bluish color, accompanied with dreadful burning pains; sensation of insects crawling over the part; great restlessness, cannot keep still in any position; excessive hyperesthesia of the part.

ANTHRAX (MALIGNANT PUSTULE)

DEFINITION—It is a specific disease followed by local and constitutional symptoms, produced by inoculation from a poison developed in the lower animals.

SYMPTOMS—Slight itching and smarting at the point of inoculation. In twenty-four hours the part becomes red, inflamed, angry looking, in the centre of which develops a large vesicle or bleb filled with a clear serum. Contents of the vesicle soon become purulent and bloody, which soon ruptures and reveals the dark gangrenous ulceration. The neighboring glands and lymphatics soon become affected, the gangrenous patch enlarges, sloughing takes place, and general infection of the whole system follows until death relieves the suffering of the patient. As the infection proceeds it is often accompanied with rigors, vomiting, great prostration, rapid pulse, profuse perspiration, and often diarrhœa, patient rapidly sinking into a typhoid state with a sudden collapse.

Pathology—The inoculation is followed by intense inflammatory reaction, serous exudations and infiltrations, thrombosis of the vesicles or hæmorrhages into internal organs.

Etiology—The virus is derived from animals, dead or suffering from splenic fever.

Diagnosis—Diagnosis is easy when we take into consideration the initial lesion, the malignancy, and the rapid development of the symptoms in the order mentioned.

Prognosis—The prognosis must be always considered grave, although under homœopathic treatment many cases recover.

Treatment—Remedies: Anthrac., Ars., Apis., Carbo veg., Carbol. ac., Lac can., Rhus tox., Pyro., Taran.; for indications, see remedies under carbuncle.

IMPETIGO

DEFINITION—An acute pustular disease of the skin, characterized by the formation of discrete, round or oval pustules, situated on a slightly inflamed base. They are little elevated above the skin, and are in size from that of a split pea to a ten cent piece.

SYMPTOMS—The disease is frequently preceded by a slight malaise and mild febrile symptoms, followed in a day or two by the pustular eruption, which appears upon the face, hands, feet and lower extremities. The contents of the pustule are of a sero-purulent nature, of a straw color, but sometimes it becomes slightly bloody. The lesions do not tend to rupture, although on pricking them a thin purulent fluid escapes. The contents, however, in a few days are absorbed, and the lesions dry up into thin, yellowish brown crusts, which in time drop off, leaving no scar.

Pathology—Inflammation involves only the papular layer of the corium. Robinson states that it is a corpuscular inflammation, the embryonic corpuscles being present in great numbers.

Etiology—It is a rare non-contagious disease, found in children who are improperly fed and cared for.

IMPETIGO CONTAGIOSA

DEFINITION—An acute inflammatory, contagious affection, characterized by the development of isolated vesicles, blebs, or vesico-pustules, which dry up into thin, yellow crusts.

SYMPTOMS—Lesions are usually few in number, generally making their appearance upon the hands and face. They are small at first, but gradually increase in size, frequently coalescing. The contents are at first transparent, then sero-purulent or purulent; if the bleb is broken a reddish, abraded-looking surface is exposed, secreting a thin puriform liquid. A few days later they dry into yellow sulphur-colored crusts. They seem loosely attached, may be single or multiple; new ones appear as the old ones disappear; they are usually accompanied with slight itching. Scratch-marks or abrasions upon the skin can be inoculated from the secretion. Sometimes the mucous membrane of the eye and nose is implicated by the production of little ulcers, similar to the lesion upon the skin.

Diagnosis—The preceding, mild febrile symptoms, its

epidemic character, the discrete vesicles, which enlarge into blebs and later on become pustular. The characteristic dry, friable, straw-colored crusts, looking as if they stuck on the skin, make the diagnosis simple. It may be confounded with eczema, impetigo simplex, ecthyma and pemphigus.

It is differentiated from pustula eczema from the fact that in eczema there is more or less infiltration and thickening of the skin, besides in eczema it is accompanied with intense itching, together with the history of the case. It differs from impetigo simplex, from the fact that the disease is pustular from the beginning. They are elevated, rounded, with the absence of tendency to flatten or to become umbilicated. It differs from ecthyma by the absence of the inflammatory base and areola; impetigo being a disease of childhood. It differs from pemphigus, from the fact that it begins with a bleb, and the absence of the constitutional symptoms.

Prognosis—Self-limiting and easily cured by constitutional treatment; no local treatment is needed.

REMEDIES—Ant. cr., Ars., Baryta carb., Cal. c., Cicuta vir., Clematis, Con., Crot. tig., Euphorb., Graph., Lyc., Mer., Mezer., Nit a., Rhus tox., Sulph., Tart. em., Viola tri., Nat mur.

INDICATIONS—*Antim. crud*—Pustules like varicella with thick, yellow crusts, tendency to coalesce; the child is cross and cannot bear to be touched, worse from bathing, tongue coated, thick, white, milky.

Arsenicum—Pale, poorly-nourished children with scrofulous tendency; the discharge from the pustule is thin and watery, and excoriates and inflames the healthy tissue it passes over.

Cicuta vir—Crusts are lemon colored, and appear

about the chin and lower portions of the face, which fall off and leave a bright red, smooth surface, accompanied with burning and itching.

Cal. carb—When the eruption appears during dentition, in large headed children, who sweat profusely about the head and face; skin pale, flabby; eruption exudes a thick, bland secretion.

Euphorbium—Small pea-sized, yellow vesicles; biting sensation in the lesions; greasy taste in the mouth, syphilitic children.

Croton tig—Eruption upon a very inflamed base, with itching and stinging pains, often appearing in the septum of the nose; pustules coalesce, crusts grayish brown; itching, burning, stinging; better by rubbing gently.

Hepar—Soft, friable crusts; excretion thin yellow pus. The lesion is very red and sensitive to touch, is worse by cold air or cold bathing; bleeds easily, abrasions on other parts of the body do not heal kindly.

Mercurius—The lesions involve the deeper layers of the epidermis; tendency to ulcerate with bloody secretions.

Rhus tox—Rheumatic or gouty patients; pustules containing a dark colored fluid burn and itch violently; stinging, tingling, better by moving about; eruption appears in clusters.

PEMPHIGUS

DEFINITION—Pemphigus is an acute or chronic disease characterized by a successive formation of irregularly scattered, variously-sized blebs.

SYMPTOMS—There are two varieties, the vulgaris and the foliaceas. The eruption is generally preceded by a slight chill or general malaise, sometimes nausea and vomiting. The temperature of two or three degrees is not uncommon. In other cases the eruption will appear without any constitutional disturbance, the blebs suddenly making their appearance, irregularly scattered about, and arising from an erythematous base, and inflamed. The blebs are tense, well formed, roundish or oval, and are from the size of that of a small pea to that of a goose egg. They contain a clear, transparent fluid, and are surrounded by an apparently healthy skin, but in some cases there may be a narrow band of erythema. The discharge gradually becomes puriform. When the blebs are not opened they gradually dry up, their exudation being absorbed; and drying up into thick brown crusts, which fall off, leaving a reddened epidermis with some pigmentation.

Successive crops of the bullæ or blebs make their appearance, and are usually attended with more or less fever.

Of its etiology or morbid anatomy nothing is known.

Prognosis—Unless the disease diverges into the foliaceous variety, or other grave forms, the prognosis is favorable.

Unless the patient receives the proper treatment the disease may last from two to six months.

Treatment—The patient should be placed upon a nourishing and easily digested diet, with plenty of fresh air, and other hygienic advantages, giving every attention to the selection of the constitutional remedy in order to bring up the patient's health to a normal standard; any of the antipsoric remedies may be indicated, but among the most frequently called for in this disease are Amm. mur., Ars., Canth., Caust., China, Dulc., Gum. gut., Hep., Hydrocotyle, Jug. cin., Lach., Lyc., Lac can., Mer. sol., Rhus tox., Phos., Sulph., Sep., Apis.

The foliaceous form is very rarely met with. The symptoms, however, are much more severe than the vulgaric form. The croupous forms are followed by fibrous exudation and even sluffing.

ECTHYMA

DEFINITION—Ecthyma is a pustular disease, characterized by the development of one or more isolated pustules upon an inflammatory base, followed by cicatrization of the skin and pigmentation.

SYMPTOMS—It begins as a pea-sized pustule, and increases in size to a dime or that of a twenty-five cent piece. They are flat, and have a marked inflammatory base and areola, accompanied with infiltration and induration of the underlying tissue. They are at first a light yellow color, but become of a reddish brown. In about a week they dry up into yellowish or reddish brown crusts, depending, of course, on the nature of the exudate. If any of these crusts are removed, the surface is found to be excoriated or ulcerated; covered with a purulent or bloody secretion. These crusts fall off in two or three weeks leaving a brown pigmentation and cicatrix. Sometimes the disease runs into a chronic state. It occurs at all ages and in both sexes.

Pathology—The disease is truly a pustular one, often of a severe nature. It is located in the upper layers of the corium.

Etiology—General debility and depraved state of the blood; met with more frequently in the lower walks of life, prisons, poor houses, slum districts. Psora, with a hereditary syphilitic taint, is probably the primary cause.

Diagnosis—It differs from impetigo by the character and size of the lesion—the marked inflammatory base being deeper seated and slower in its progress.

Prognosis—Prognosis good.

Treatment—Treatment consists in the removal of the acting miasm, as presented in totality of the symptoms, together with the betterment of the patient's sanitary surroundings, fresh air and good food.

Arsenic—Red pustules on a marked inflammatory base with much burning. Pale cachetic patients who suffer from general debility and lack of strength, and who are generally better from warmth.

Asafoetida—Nervous patients with a history of latent or tertiary syphilis; lesions sensitive, hard edges, bleed easily; pus profuse, greenish, thin, ichorous and very offensive.

Carbo veg—Dark, black looking pustules, scorbutic, livid, fetid, burning at night.

Hepar—Scrofulous individuals with marked tubercular or latent syphilitic taint; profuse yellowish pus secretion. Lesions sensitive to touch and to cold air, with dread of being uncovered.

Mercurius—Dark, bloody pustules with a very red, angry base, bleeding easily, tendency to ulcerate; bloody pus exudes from under the dark, thick crusts; worse at night and from warmth; sweats profusely, which is musty or offensive—giving no relief.

Rhus tox—Black pustules seated upon a very dark inflammatory base, filled at first with a straw colored serum; later on bloody, pustules burn and itch, worse at night and with every change of weather. Sycotic patients.

Sulphur—Dry, thick, yellow crusts, more especially on the scalp, accompanied with much itching, smarting and burning after scratching or rubbing, which is increased by warmth.

Kali bich—Indicated in light-haired, fleshy children, chubby or short-necked individuals, who are subject to laryngeal and croupous affections. Thick, yellow-coated tongue, pustules resembling small-pox; skin dry, hot, very red, discharge stringy or ropy.

Petroleum—Itching, burning pustules, painful to touch, better by warmth; lesions bleed easily, crusts moist, friable, purulent secretion; all the symptoms better in the summer.

PRURIGO

DEFINITION—A papular eruption confined to some part of the skin, or extending over the whole surface, accompanied with intense and constant itching, generally assuming a chronic form.

SYMPTOMS—Prurigo is a rare disease in this country, comprising probably less than one per cent. of all diseases of the skin. It differs from pruritus, from the fact that in pruritus there is no visible alteration in the skin and that prurigo is followed by pigmentation. It appears from the sixth to twelfth month of infant life, first as a sort of urticaria, or by the presence of a few scattered millet-seed sized papules, slightly elevated above the skin. It is worse upon the extensor surfaces, the tibia being a favorite seat. In the beginning the skin is dry, rough, harsh; itching is intense, and the result of scratching forms crust, pustules and thickening of the skin. It may last for years and is difficult to cure.

Pathology—It is probably a true neurosis or a neurotic disturbance in the papillary layer of the corium.

Etiology—It is undoubtedly of psoric origin, as all diseases where pruritus is marked are of a psoric nature. It attacks those children whose health is below normal.

Diagnosis—A careful study of the papillary lesion, together with a dry, harsh skin, with the pale face, and the other clinical symptoms.

6

Prognosis—Guarded until a remedy can be selected to meet the psoric taint, when it must disappear.

Treatment—Study indications of remedies under pruritus.

ECZEMA (Salt Rheum, Tetter, Crusta Lac)

DEFINITION—(*To boil over*). An acute or chronic inflammatory, non-contagious disease of the skin, polymorphic in its nature, appearing in one or more of the elementary lesions.

FORMS—Erythematous, papular, pustular, vesicular, fissum, and nodosum. It also receives its name from its anatomical location, as facial eczema capitis, etc.

Eczema may have for its basis any of the chronic miasms, but probably no other disease gives a fuller and clearer conception of the profound and persistent action of psora, as does eczema, presenting itself as it does in both sexes and in all ages, from the infant of a few days old to that of old age. Few diseases have the pruritus of eczema so characteristic of psora. Its multiplicity of forms and the innumerable variety of its phenomena, besides the frequency with which it makes its appearance, gives it, probably, the foremost place of interest and study to the dermatologists of this country.

Symptomatology—The symptoms of this disease can only be studied separately under each form; even then only a typical case may be studied, as seldom two cases present exactly the same phenomena, yet their difference of aspect is, as we will see, due more to the dissimilarity of the lesions, which can be almost alphabetically combined. Besides a tubercular, syphilitic, or sycotic diathesis multiplies this dissimilarity of lesions.

Eczema Erythematosum—The erythema is a constant

symptom, yet many of the other lesions may complicate the disease. It begins with a slight tingling or formication over a smaller or greater surface of the skin. This, of course, induces rubbing or scratching, which is followed by the erythematous patch, the color of which may be bright red or any variation, even to a yellowish tinge. Minute vesicles or papules may be seen upon the surface. There is slight swelling, depending largely upon the anatomical location. Later on the surface assumes a hard, rough feeling, or becomes covered with scales. A feeling of tension is not uncommon accompanied with more or less itching, with slight, if any, moisture. It is a disease prone to relapses and to run into a chronic state. It is found more frequently in middle age or in old people.

ECZEMA PUSTULOSUM

This form of eczema may begin as a pustule or it may develop from either the erythematous, vesicular, or papular forms. It is more frequently associated with the vesicular form, and it is often quite difficult to distinguish which was the primary lesion. The vesicles fill with a purulent secretion, which from over-distension or from any irritation break and pour out a profuse purulent matter, which soon dries into a greenish yellow, or dark colored crust. A raw, sensitive surface is exposed by the breaking off of one of these friable crusts. The discharge may become ichorous and inflamed, or irritate the surrounding tissue.

The local symptoms are heat, swelling, itching, tenderness, and soreness, and in some cases it is often accompanied with marked infiltration. Should the hairy scalp become affected and the sebaceous glands involved, the discharges then become mixed with a granular secretion, the hair matted together, and large crusts form from this purulent secretion and excrementitious matter, which soon becomes rancid and, of course, very offensive. This form of eczema appears in strumous or tubercular children, frequently upon the scalp, and is sometimes called seborrheic eczema.

ECZEMA VESICULOSUM

SYMPTOMS—Vesicular eczema begins with sensation of heat accompanied with a slight pruritus, which is rapidly followed by a localized congestion, and within a few hours often the whole erythematous field is covered with fine vesicles filled with a transparent lymph fluid; rubbing or scratching soon destroys them, and they pour out their secretion over the whole diseased surface. This discharge is of alkaline reaction, plastic in its nature, and on drying up forms thin crusts, which may be light or dark in color. Other lesions may be present, more especially the papular and pustular. This form of eczema appears probably more frequently upon the face or hands of either children or adults, but it may occur upon any part of the body, more frequently in irritable and nervous subjects. It disappears gradually, leaving the skin red, sensitive and tender to touch. Relapses are prone to occur, and the disease often passes into a chronic state (eczema rubrum). Where the crusts dry up and it disappears by desquamation when it is called eczema squamosum.

PAPULOSUM

The forms of eczema that we have previously considered have had as a characteristic feature some form of exudate, but in the papular form we find the surface comparatively dry. As an initial symptom some form of hyperesthesia of the affected part is present, which is followed by an eruption, papular in form, usually of a pin-head size. They may be close together, or appreciably separated. The pruritus accompanying the appearance of the papules induces scratching when the tops of the papules are torn off, and the small quantity of lymph that exudes dries into minute scales. In the course of time the disease subsides, leaving no scar or pigmentation. Its favorite seat is on the arms, forearms, legs, and flexure surfaces.

ECZEMA FISSUM

This is a chronic form found in patients of a tubercular taint. It is typically a manifestation of latent syphilis upon a psoric base. The patients are usually free from it during the dry, hot summer months, suffering relapses from the disease usually in the fall and spring. It is prone to occur in prolonged wet or snowy weather, especially if there is much moisture in the atmosphere. It is aggravated by cold, wet weather and working in water. It affects those parts where the epidermis is thickest, as on the hands and feet, flexure surfaces of the joints, lips, corners of the mouth, face, and behind the ears. The slightest irritation of the skin in these patients often produces it, such as the handling of irritants, exposure to various kinds of weather, the excessive use of water or soap; dyers, wool pickers, masons, plasterers, outdoor laborers, etc., are prone to this disease. The skin becomes dry, harsh, very much thickened and fissured. The fissures are mechanically induced by the flexing of the skin in its dry, hard, and thickened condition, which is, of course, due to inflammatory changes. The fissures are sometimes quite superficial; again they may extend deeply into the corium, showing raw, tender, and bleeding surfaces. Frequently they may be accompanied with erythematous patches, and usually with more or less pruritus. The surface may remain dry or there may be more or less oozing of a sticky honey-like secretion, and often bleeding from the deeper fissure.

ECZEMA RUBRUM

This is the severest form of this disease. It may result from either the erythematous, vesicular, pustular, or papular forms. It is characterized by a reddened, hot, tumefied, weeping surface. At times it is covered with sero-purulent exudation. The epidermis may be entirely denuded, and the exposed corium pour forth serum or an ichorous, bloody secretion which dries into crusts, often covering the whole diseased surface. It usually takes on a chronic character, marked infiltration follows, and the parts become hardened, thickened, and rough, showing no tendency to a spontaneous cure. It is found more frequently in the flexures of the body, joints, nates, groin, etc. In infants it frequently appears upon the face and scalp, and upon the lower extremities of people of advanced years.

Pathology—Eczema is essentially an inflammation of the skin, situate chiefly in the rete and papillary layer; in prolonged chronic cases it may affect the lower layer of the corium and even the connective tissue. The vascular changes are the same as observed in all inflammations, edematous swelling, diapedesis of white blood cells, and a plentiful serous exudation.

Diagnosis—Diagnosis is made easy, if we take into consideration the history of the case, the multiple lesions and their progress as observed by the patient. The exudation and mode of crusting can hardly be similarly met with in other diseases. It is to be distinguished from erysipelas, psoriasis, seborrhea, sycosis, scabies, and ring-worm.

Prognosis—The prognosis is favorable in infant, childhood, and adult life, up to fifty years; after that age it is sometimes difficult to eradicate. As a disease, above all others, it is prone to relapses and recurrences. But the majority of cases are curable where a careful individualization is made and a thorough study of the miasmatic basis in each case.

Treatment—Eczema is always of constitutional origin, and the patient, as well as the physician, should be well pleased to know that the life force had divorced it from within and thrown it as an eczematous eruption upon the skin. We have the worst forms to deal with in the tubercular or syphilitic child, especially during the teething period. No man can tell how many of these little lives are saved, by the disease coming to the surface, preserving the vital organs, especially the brain, from the ravages of this destructive miasm; therefore, all ointments and medicants of every name and description are to be discarded *in toto;* depending alone upon the anti-miasmatic treatment or the removal of the miasm which alone is the pre-disposing cause; using by preference the higher potencies. Not repeating often, but giving the life force plenty of time for their free action. The author never uses any local measures in any disease of the skin except it be heat, sweet or pure olive oil as a lubricant. The pruritus of eczema, which is so positively a psoric symptom, is the flag of distress for the life force, and its removal by the well-selected remedy is a pretty sure sign you have reached down to the miasmatic basis of the disease.

The vocation, diet and habits of the patient are first in

importance for consideration; especially is this true as to diet in the treatment of young children; and more in particular with bottle-fed babies, a change of diet will frequently work wonders in this disease. Keep them in the fresh air as much as possible, and while bathing is not to be neglected, however, too much bathing is, as a rule, harmful, as all diseases of the skin are rebellious to water.

REMEDIES—Acon., Bell., Dulc., Phosp., Plat., Pb., Puls., Par., Agar., Ang., Alum., Amm. carb., Amm. mur., Anac., Ant. cr., Ant. t., Arg., Arn., Ars., Asaf., Asar, Aur., Bary. c., Bary. m., Bism., Bor., Bov., Calad., Calc., Canth., Cap., Carb. v., Caust., Cham., Chel., Chin., Cic., Clem., Colch., Coloc., Con., Croc., Cup., Fer., Graph., Hep., Iod., Kali c., Kali bi., Kali nit., Kali pho., Lach., Lyc., Led., Mag. c., Meny., Merc., Mez., Nat. c., Nat. m., Nit. ac., Nux v., Olea., Op., Petrol., Rhodo., Rhus, Ruta, Sabina, Samb., Sars., Sep., Sul., Sil., Stan., Staph., Thuj., Viol., Zinc., Psor., Syph., Tubercul., Medorrh., X-ray, Teuc., Tell., Crot. tig., Lac can., Bacc., Ham., Hyd.

INDICATIONS—*Alumina*, Bil. mot. temp. Spare, dry, thin subjects, dark complected with mild, cheerful disposition, latent syphilitic patients, who suffer with dry, tettery, itching eruptions that are worse in winter; itching worse when warm in bed, scratches until it bleeds, when it becomes painful, craves starch, chalk, charcoal, indigestible things; habitual constipation.

Anacardium—Dark red, erythematous eruption, covered with little vesicles (Rhus), red spots like urticaria, eruptions go from right to left; excoriation of the epidermis; erysipelatous-like eruption, swelling with burning of the parts; miliary pustules, bad tempered people who are inclined to swear.

Ant. tart—Shrivelled, dry skin; erythematous eruptions of the hands and face; itching pustules that soon dry up; pustular eruptions above the nose and face; vesicles all over the body which quickly fill with pus and dry up into crusts; umbilicated pustules, similar to vaccination or small-pox; pea-sized pustules which leave a scar or a bluish red mark; white, pasty-coated tongue; great dread of touch; large blisters filled with serum. It is indicated after bad effects of vaccination, pustular eczema with dark thick crusts.

Apis—The erythematous eruption shows swelling and marked edema (complementary to Nat. mur.), not to be given after Rhus; eruptions worse on the face, lips, nose, ears, throat, hands, and feet; circumscribed spots that itch, burn and sting; skin often swollen, edematous, pale, waxy, or dirty looking; deep red rash or dark red papules; worse in a warm room and better by bathing and open air.

Arsenicum—San. bil. ment. Deep chronic cases; skin like parchment, dry, rough, or dirty looking; child usually emaciated and suffering with some other deep chronic trouble. Squama, thin, white bran-like (Nat. mur.) vesicles, small, transparent, secreting a thin, watery exudation that excoriates the parts passed over; all eruptions itch intensely and are accompanied with burning and smarting; discharge usually offensive; better by warm applications or heat in general.

Aurum—Sang. or bil. nerv. temp. Ruddy people with black hair and eyes; lively, restless, anxious about the future; constitutions broken down from the bad effects of mercury or from syphilis. It is followed well by Syphilinum. Dark yellow skin, itching worse by warmth; eczema worse in the summer.

Agaricus—Eczema with burning, itching, pricking as

from needles; electric-like stitches in the skin; small nodules deep in the skin; eczema worse in the winter and accompanied with chilblains; bright red erythema with burning, biting, tingling, and intense itching.

Ammonium mur—Eruptions in the flexures of the joints, about the anus, thighs, sexual organs; burning and rawness of the affected part; vesicular eczema with tension and burning in the part; relieved by hot bathing. It is indicated in fat, sluggish people, with large bodies and thin legs.

Baryta carb—Sang. lymp. temp. Tubercular diathesis, dwarfish children, who suffer with glandular enlargement; eczema of old people and drunkards. It is often followed well by Tub., Psor., Syph. Intolerable itching and tingling; worse by scratching and by thinking about it; parts red, excoriated, accompanied with much burning; erythematous eczema in the folds and flexures of the body.

Borax—Very sycotic children with wilted, wrinkled, dry skin; light-haired children who suffer with aphthæ during dentition, and have a constant dread of falling; eruption dark red, erysipelatous-like; scaly patches similar to psoriasis.

Bovista—Sang. lymp. temp. Moist vesicular eruptions with formation of thick crusts, no relief from scratching; eruptions may be dry or moist; rough, dark red, moist eczema in the bends of the knees, appearing during the full moon. It is indicated more frequently in women who suffer from dysmenorrhea.

Cal. carb—Sang. lymp. temp. Blonde, blue-eyed, fair skinned, pale, weak, easily-tired women or children; chubby, fat babies who are deficient in bone with an excess of flesh; large headed children with pale skin, soft, flabby muscles and who are self-willed; cold, clammy hands and feet; eruptions either dry or moist; yellowish thick crusts in seborrheic eczema of the scalp; latent syphilitic diathesis; discharges light yellow, offensive, puslike. Location: scalp, face, behind the ears, forearm.

Cal. phos—Bil. mot. temp. Anæmic, dark complexioned people, dark hair and eyes, scrofulous children, who are emaciated, weak and unable to stand alone; dry crusty affections; tubercular eczema, injured parts become the seat of eczematous eruptions. Constitutional symptoms are the only safe guide in this remedy.

Causticum—Yellowish looking skin; eczema about the wings of the nose. Pustular eczema with burning and biting, preventing sleep.

Cicuta vir—Sang. or bil. nerv. temp. Pustules which run together, forming thick, yellow crusts; suppurating eczema, which dries into hard, lemon colored crusts; scaly, moist, itchy eruption on the scalp; light complexioned blue-eyed children who are subject to convulsions.

Clematis—Vesicular and pustular eczema, with purulent or watery secretion, followed by a formation of scales and crusts, which are inflamed during the increasing, and dry during the decrease of the moon; dark, rough, firmly adhering crusts upon the scalp, exuding a yellowish excoriating fluid; itching worse by warmth; eruption often follows, suppressed sycosis.

Colchicum—Eczema rubrum in old people, beer or wine drinkers, accompanied with a marked uric acid or lithic condition of the system. The eczema increases or decreases with the inactivity of the liver or the gouty condition. Eczema of the face, nose, forehead, accompanied with hot, highly colored, scanty urination and rheumatic or gouty symptoms.

Dulcamara—Bil. mot. temp. Phlegmatic, scrofulous

constitutions. Vesicular eruptions on red, inflamed base, oozing a watery fluid. Impetiginous eczema of scrofulous children, who suffer with glandular enlargements; itching worse by warmth, from washing, better by cold, worse in the winter and by cold and wet weather.

Graphites—Sang. lymp. temp. Indicated in blondes who are inclined to obesity and habitual constipation.

The eczema is often accompanied with erysipelas; patients who never perspire, who normally have a thin, sensitive skin, who are always suffering with chapped hands; skin dry, greatly thickened, rough, horny, fissured, deep cracks that bleed easily or exude a watery, sticky fluid. Eczema with profuse, serous exudation; worse by wet or in snowy weather. The favorite seats of the eruptions are on the hands, face, lips, behind the ears, joints and flexures of the body (Tub., Petr., Psor., Hep., Teuc.).

Hepar—Sang. lymp. temp. Pustular and erythematous forms of eczema in torpid lymphatic constitutions, persons with light hair and complexion, soft, flabby muscles, who are slow to act, who are extremely sensitive to cold; croupy children, who perspire profusely; with unhealthy skin, slightest injury heals unkindly. Eczema often spreads by new papules appearing on the outer surface of the patch. Eczema with profuse yellowish discharge and the parts very sensitive to touch; lesions red, raw, bleeding easily, sensitive to cold and to touch and bathed with a profuse yellowish purulent secretion; pustular or seborrheic eczema with soft, friable, yellow crusts, oozing a yellow pus, smelling like old cheese.

Iris ver—Pustular or vesicular eczema accompanied with great itching, especially at night, or vesicular eruptions becoming pustular. Eczema with gastric complaints.

Juglans—Large, thickly-set confluent pustules, worse on the hands and arms, secretion ichorous, producing sores upon the healthy skin. Eczematous patches have a tendency to coalesce. Pustules discharge and crust over, and are accompanied with tension or with unbearable pain about them. One crop of pustules hardly subsides before another appears. Indicated in very psoric patients.

Lycopodium—Eruptions first vesicular then dry, humid, suppurating, full of deep rhagades. Eczema of the face, genitals, any part of the body, covered with thick crusts, or bleeding easily, moist, scald head, or moisture behind the ears; eruptions have great tendency to ulcerate, itching worse at night while in bed; much belching with gastric disturbances.

Lachesis—Eczema of the erythematous pustular vesicular and nodosus forms. Left-sided eczema dark bluish, erythema very sensitive to slightest touch, dark bluish vesicular eruptions, burning itching with formication like ants, pruritus intense, almost driving the patient to distraction, worse after sleep; parts very red and swollen and sensitive; bluish colored pustules with red streaks along the lymphatic vessels.

Mercur. sol.—Eczema of the chest, forearms and legs; yellow crusts with inflamed areola; pustules exuding bloody, purulent secretion; skin dirty yellow, rough and dry, scaly; itching intolerable; worse at night, by warmth of bed; better in the daytime and by cold; eruption has tendency to ulceration, to bleed easily and is frequently copper colored.

Mezereum—Eczema rubrum in latent syphilitic patients, thick crusts oozing a bloody, purulent secretion, itching worse at night and by warmth; cold skin covered with white scabs; bleeds easily when touched.

6

Natrum mur—Fine vesicular eruption all over the body, with intense itching that is worse by cold air and undressing; vesicles dry up, leaving a thin crust. Eczema raw inflamed, discharging a corrosive fluid, worse in edges of hair, genitals, bends of the joints and flexure surfaces; low-spirited, despondent people with tubercular taint who crave salt and sour things.

Petroleum—Eczema dry, scaly or moist, disappearing in the summer and reappearing in the winter or cold weather. Like Hepar, the slightest wound causes suppuration. Eczema fissure occurring on the hands or behind the ears, a moist, purulent secretion, usually offensive, and bleeding easily; pustules burn and itch; eczema often accompanied with chilblains; aggravation in the morning and in open air; itching and burning often accompanied with chilliness.

Psorinum—Eruption dry and scaly, moist or suppurating; low-spirited, despondent, unhopeful patients who dread the cold; skin dry, dirty looking; eczema of the scalp, bends and flexures of the body, behind the ears; in pale, peevish, delicate children; discharges thin, fetid, excoriating; itching worse in the evening and the open air; better by warmth and by rest.

Rhus tox—Sang.. mot. temp. Dark erythematous eruption more or less vesicular, thin, watery, dark colored and quite offensive secretion; hardness and thickening of the skin; dark, thin brown crusts; intense burning and itching; vesicles often contain a yellowish or straw colored serum; location of eruption usually on the scalp, race, hands, lower extremities, genitals; itching worse by warmth, better by motion and rubbing.

Sepia—Dark complexioned, dark haired, delicate skinned people. Eczema accompanied with pelvic or uterine disturbances; the lesions usually take on a brownish pigmentation, or eruptions alternate with uterine affections; are worse during or after menstruation. Eruptions often assume a circular form or appear in rings; better by warmth; eruption worse in the flexures of the joints, dry, scaly, brownish patches.

Sulphur—Sang. ment. mot. temp. Deeply psoric patients with dry, pimply skin, who never perspire; discharges usually scanty, frequently bloody; all eruptions accompanied with intense itching, which is worse at night and by warmth of bed; scratching relieves the itching but is followed by burning and smarting, scratches until it bleeds; stoop-shouldered patients who dread to stand or to take a bath, who suffer from hot feet and from an empty, gone feeling in the stomach between ten and eleven o'clock, relieved by eating; imperfectly developed or suppressed eruptions.

Tellurium—Eruptions spread in circles or rings accompanied with itching, prickling, stinging sensations that are worse in the evening.

Syphilinum—Eczema following tertiary or latent syphilis, especially the pustular forms; pus yellowish green, thick, ichorous, offensive; crusts dark green even black, with oozing of ichorous, bloody pus; dry, scaly, brown or copper colored eruptions; brown, scaly patches in the bends of the elbows and flexures of the body; many cases cured; follows Sepia well; itching only slight; eruptions worse in summer; indicated in blonde, absent-minded people who have very little energy.

Viola tri—Impetiginoid eczema on a scrofulous base; milk crusts of children, with miliary eruptions all over the body; crusts on the face, with burning pruritus, worse at night; exudation yellow, viscous pus with swelling of the cervical glands.

Thuja—Sang. lymp. temp. Sycotic patients, or after suppressed gonorrhea; eczema following vaccination, dirty brown skin, covered with itching vesicles; eruptions worse on covered parts; moles and warty growths scattered over the body, white, scaly, measly eruption; biting, stinging after scratching; follows Medorrhinum in suppressed gonorrhea.

X-Ray—Dark blue erythematous eruption, resembling a burn, deep cracks and fissures in the hands and feet, knees and extensor surface of the joints; very deep fissures (Kali, Iod., Pel., Tub., Graph). Erysipelatous eruptions, or skin dry, scaly, cracked; much swelling of the part, with smarting, burning and intense itching; milk crusts in children about the face. It antidotes the overuse of sulphur.

Tuberculinum—Sang. mot. temp. Adapted to light complected people with blue eyes, tall, slim, flat narrow chested, with a family history of tubercular affections; melancholy; despondent; morose; takes cold easily, always chilly; symptoms ever changing, tubercular eruptions with greenish pus; oozing behind the ears, fiery red skin with rawness and soreness in folds of the skin; eczema over the entire body, itching worse at night, intense when undressing (Nat. mur., Ars., Hep.).

DERMATITIS SEBORRHOICA

Definition—An erythematous form of seborrhea of a catarrhal nature usually situated in the scalp.

Symptoms—The disease usually begins in the scalp and in the region of the vertex, and generally extending to the ears, face and sometimes other parts of the body. It follows sometimes a slow and at other times a rapid course, and when well established remains stationary for months or years. The lesions may be discrete, or closely run together. The squamæ is abundant, white or yellowish brown in color, elevated slightly in patches, and covered more or less with greasy scales. When the scales are removed, it presents a raw surface, and sometimes a slight oozing takes place. Itching of mild nature exists, especially when the patient becomes heated. Sometimes the scales, owing to the fatty matter, present a granular appearance. The hair is dry, lustreless and dirty looking; a form of this disease sometimes affects the eyelids, showing slight scaling and crusting; their borders become red and swollen. The disease may exist alone or with some other disease.

Etiology—The disease occurs between the ages of ten and thirty years, and in both sexes alike. It is also worse in cold weather.

Diagnosis—The disease differs from pityriasis maculata from the fact that it does not follow the same method of extension, and that it is limited mostly to the trunk and extremities, while the seborrheic is limited to the scalp, and they are larger and fawn colored; besides there is much itching.

Treatment—Consult remedies under eczema and psoriasis.

PITYRIASIS MACULATA ET CIRCINATA

Symptomatology—This form of pityriasis is an erythematous disease consisting of rose colored macules of different sizes, round or oval; usually, slightly elevated above the skin, and covered with greasy scales. There are no premonitory symptoms to speak of. The first notice of the disease is generally the appearance of the eruption. The spots are from the size of a ten-cent piece to that of a silver dollar, confined closely to the trunk.
7

The macules gradually increase in size and number. The eruption is dry throughout, and lasts from six to eight weeks, gradually fading out in the order they come.

Pathology—Mild hyperemia of the papillary layer of the derma, with slight exudation and scaling.

Etiology—Nothing is known.

HERPES

DEFINITION—From the Greek meaning "to creep." It is an acute, non-contagious, inflammatory disease, characterized by groups or clusters of vesicles on a reddened base. Four forms may be mentioned: Herpes simplex, herpes facialis or febrilis, herpes progenitalis, herpes zoster.

Herpes Simplex—Herpes simplex is characterized by one or more groups of vesicles on a reddened base and running a typical course, distinguished from the facialis only by its location.

Herpes Facialis—Hydroa or herpes febrilis, commonly known as cold sore or fever blisters.

SYMPTOMS—It appears upon any part of the face, the lips being the more favored point of attack. The vesicles are small, few in number, usually in groups, but they may be isolated; sometimes they involve the mucous membrane of the nose, mouth, and tongue. They may follow a cold, fever, menstrual irregularity, malarial conditions, rheumatism, or acute febrile states. They consist of small transparent vesicles filled with clear serum, and situated on a reddened base.

Pathology—It is supposed to be a neurotic disturbance, probably reflex in its nature.

Diagnosis—History of the case, the transparent vesicles, their location and their short duration, with no tendency to crust.

Prognosis—Prognosis is good.

Treatment—Based upon the constitutional symptoms if possible.

Remedies—Acon., Bell., Ars., Bry., Rhus tox, Nat. mur., Hep., Merc., Nat. carb., Sepia, Puls., Sulph.

Herpes Progenitalis—Symptomatology: It consists in an eruption of grouped vesicles about the genital organs. In men the most common seat is on the glands and preputial surface. In women it invades most frequently the labia, clitoris, vestibule, perineum, and external genital surfaces. The first symptoms are slight burning or itching followed by an eruption of pin-head-sized vesicles closely grouped together on an inflamed base; slight edema and swelling; later on the vesicles rupture, leaving circumscribed, grayish-white, raw spots. If properly cared for they disappear in a few days, leaving no scar; sometimes they ulcerate and may be taken for a chancre.

Diagnosis—The importance of the diagnosis in these cases is clearly evident. In the vesicular stage there is no difficulty; it is, however, quite difficult if ulceration takes place. The decisive points, however, are their quick appearance, the arrangement of the vesicular group, their short course and a tendency to quick recovery. In chancroid there is a destructive tendency, while in chancre there is the induration and sympathetic involvement of the glands. The treatment is simple and consists in proper bathing, cleanliness and the indicated remedy.

Herpes Zoster—Definition: Meaning "a belt." An acute typical inflammatory disease of the skin, appearing in the course of certain cutaneous nerves, accompanied by severe neuralgic pain, and by the presence of groups of firm, tense vesicles rising from an edematous base.

Symptoms—The disease may be ushered in by general

malaise and febrile symptoms, but frequently it begins with stitching pains in the region of the affected part. Pain is generally sharp, but may be dull and heavy. The favorite location of the disease is about the sides or chest. The pains are of a neuralgic character, appearing often days before the appearance of the eruption, and usually aggravated by respiration. The eruption begins in reddened or bluish-red patches, which are very tender and sensitive to touch. Red papules form on its surface, which change into vesicles filled with a transparent or straw colored serum. They have very little tendency to rupture. Later on the contents may become purulent. The eruption may occur on any part of the body, but by preference it attacks the thoracic, intercostal and abdominal regions. The disease may run a mild or severe course, lasting from one to three weeks. Relapse is not infrequent. Hæmorrhagic and gangrenous forms sometimes occur, but they are very rare. The disease is apt to be of a more severe nature if it attacks the left side than the right, especially in the region of the stomach or the heart.

Pathology—Barensprung demonstrated that the disease was one of the ganglionic system. This has been confirmed by others. Cases of death, the nerves between the brain and the ganglion are surrounded by extravasated blood, the interstitial tissue of the gasserian ganglion infiltrated with inflammatory products, the intercostal nerves reddened and thickened.

Etiology—The lesion is produced by an inflammation of the nerves supplying the part. The inflammation may occur at any point in the track of the nerve, or in the ganglion through which the nerve passes. Tuberculosis with transmitted or acquired sycosis is probably the true origin of the disease.

Prognosis—Prognosis usually quite favorable. Relapses, however, may prolong the case.

Treatment—Remedies: Acon., Bell., Ars., Bry., Rhus tox., Canth., Crot. tigl., Mez., Puls., Ran. bul., Comocladia, Apis, Lach., Lac can., Phos.

INDICATIONS—*Arsenicum*—Confluent, herpetic eruptions with intense burning of the blisters. Herpes with fine scales over them, burning worse at night; thirst and the common symptoms of Arsenic.

Arsen. hydr—Dark brown, sallow, or bronze colored skin. Herpes filled with dark red blood.

Bovista—Moist or dry herpes; itching on getting warm and continued after scratching; red, scabby eruptions in the bends of the knees, appearing in hot weather and with the full moon.

Calc. carb—Pale, dry, flabby skin, bloated appearance of the skin; burning herpes; itching herpes between the fingers; herpes on disappearing, leave a raw spot; herpes in scrofulous children with enlarged glands.

Cantharis—Large herpes, like blebs, accompanied with severe pain and burning, worse in the open air and when touched; the blebs swell and exude much serum; herpes with irritation of the bladder.

Cicuta—Scaly, moist, itching eruption upon the scalp; herpes of the scalp, chin and beard, which dry into yellow crusts, matting the hair together and accompanied with burning.

Clematis—Herpes that increase during the increasing, and dry up during the decreasing of the moon; red, inflamed, moist herpes, with intolerable itching in the warmth of bed and after washing.

Croton tigl—Herpes with burning, stinging and great redness of the skin, which quickly develop a sero-purulent exudation; herpes, especially on the abdomen, becoming confluent and drying into large, dark crusts; intense itching of the part, but so tender you cannot scratch it, better by gentle rubbing.

Dulcamara—Moist suppurating herpes; herpes with a red areola; herpes drying into thick, brown crusts, occurring on the scalp, face, forehead and chin; worse in warmth and better by cold.

Graphites—Large vesicles with transparent, glutinous exudation; herpes, especially on the face, tibia; herpes zoster on the left side.

Hepar—White blisters on the lips, chin and face; humid herpes of the face filled with transparent water, which becomes purulent; base inflamed, very sensitive to touch, and bleeds easily, accompanied with burning, itching, sometimes throbbing or pricking sensation; frequently indicated in scrofulous children who are sensitive to cold.

Lachesis—All kinds of herpetic eruptions; large, of a yellow color at first, but soon turn dark, very painful and sensitive to touch; worse on the left side of the body and after sleep.

Natrum mur—Fever blisters following colds, menses, or malarial conditions; fever blisters like pearls about the lips; cracks in the corners of the mouth; herpes in the bends of the knees, moist and oozing; herpes zoster; blebs containing clear water.

Iris vers—Herpes following gastric derangements and liver troubles; herpes zoster on the right side of the body, fine vesicles showing black points, itching worse at night.

Petroleum—Herpes of the genitals, moist, oozing, worse in open air, better by warmth; herpes followed by ulcers, moist, sore or deep cracks.

Rhus tox—Pea-sized vesicles filled with a yellowish, watery fluid, accompanied with intense itching and burning, appearing in clusters with or without erythematous base; herpes zoster with dark red swelling; straw-colored vesicles that burn and itch intensely, and accompanied with marked rheumatic pains; better by motion, heat, and rubbing the part gently or by extension.

Apis—Large transparent vesicles accompanied with much swelling and stinging; burning, stinging pains, worse from warmth and better from cold applications.

MILIARIA RUBRA (Prickly Heat, Lichen Tropicus)

DEFINITION—An acute erythematous pruritus, occurring in the heat of summer, due to an obstruction of sweat-gland ducts in the lower corneal layer.

Symptomatology—It appears suddenly without any premonitory symptoms, following a hearty meal, overheating, over-exertion, etc. The eruption is characterized by the appearance of a great number of accuminated, minute, mustard-seed sized papules, situated upon a reddened base, and accompanied with more or less itching, stinging and burning in the skin. The papules are situated around the orifices of the sudoriparous ducts and are slightly elevated above the skin. They appear more frequently upon the scalp, neck, chest, back and arms. There is usually a marked increased perspiration. Sometimes the eruption is complicated by minute vesicles. It usually runs its course in a few days, terminating by absorption and desquamation.

Diagnosis—It may be mistaken for eczema papulosum, but its sudden appearance during very warm weather, the increased perspiration, the stinging, prickling and burning sensation, besides their ephemeral character and their sudden disappearance on removing the exciting cause, make the diagnosis clear.

Pathology—Hyperemia of the vessels of the sudoriparous glands; if the secretion is scant, only the papular eruption appears, but if very profuse, the vesicular also. When the hyperemia subsides the eruption absorbs and disappears.

Etiology—Exposure to undue heat, in warm climates, and improper dressing in weak and anæmic persons or corpulent children.

Treatment—Proper clothing and frequent bathing, with moderately cold or tepid water, together with regulation of the diet, rest and the remedy indicated in pruritus. For remedies see pruritus.

MILIUM

Synonym—Acne miliaria.

Definition—Milium is a small, pearly white, pin-head sized formation beneath the epidermis.

Symptoms—They appear on the face, neck, upper eyelids, cheek, and temples more frequently, although they may occur on any part of the body. They vary in size from a pin-head to a pea, may or may not be elevated. They are hard and firm to touch, whitish or yellowish in color, and appear singly or multiple; develop slowly, and after reaching a certain size remain for years. They occur more frequently in women than in men, appearing frequently after adult age.

Diagnosis—Distinguished by their anatomical formation as a very small sebaceous tumor covered with epidermis.

Pathology—Retention of the sebaceous secretion with probable calcification.

Etiology—The origin of the disease is unknown. I have, however, found them only in the tubercular or latent syphilitic patient.

DERMATITIS EXFOLIATA

DEFINITION—A sub-acute or chronic inflammation of the skin, coming on as a primary or as a secondary manifestation characterized by an intense hyperemia of the part, and followed by copious and repeated exfoliation of different sized scales, also followed by atrophy of the cutaneous appendages, with more or less complete shedding of the hair and nails.

SYMPTOMS—When the disease begins as a primary affection it is frequently ushered in by a marked chill, malaise, anorexia with nausea and vomiting. Often the symptoms are accompanied with an intense formication of the skin previous to the development of a diffuse erythematous eruption resembling erysipelas. It may, however, appear in scaly patches, bullous, or papular spots. The disease is accompanied with a tingling sensation or slight itching, the skin being sensitive to cold or the friction of the clothing.

The eruption may appear on one or more parts of the body at the same time, occurring more frequently on the lower extremities, and beginning as a small patch, the redness rapidly extending until within a few days a large portion of the integument becomes involved, the parts becoming deeply hyperemic, slightly thickened; the color from a bright red to a dark red, even to a violet hue. A temperature from a 101 to 102 and even higher may be present. The skin assumes a deeper tint, becomes lustreless; finally, in a week or two, the epidermis shrivels and comes off in large flakes.

These flakes vary in size in different patients, are larger on the back, often from one to two inches in length. On the face, however, they appear as a fine branny desquamation. On the scalp the hair often becomes matted and tangled, due to the collection of scales and sebum, as the disease involves the sebaceous glands. The exfoliation from the whole body may exceed a pint in twenty-four hours. As the layers of flakes scale off the underlying skin appears smooth and shining. Repeated exfoliations of the skin, however, take place before resolution sets in. The palms of the hands and soles of the feet are the last to be affected. The nails become opaque or of a brownish color, fissured, brittle, easily broken and often cast off.

The disease may run into a chronic state, lasting for months, even years, alternating with periods of improvement and apparent recovery, only to be followed by relapses. In the beginning the general health of the patient is not much impaired, but later on constipation alternating with diarrhœa is a pretty constant symptom; the appetite is often greatly increased, while renal complications are apt to develop; the urine being usually deficient in area, but loaded with urates; inflammations of the mucous membranes are quite common, such as conjunctivitis, stomatitis, etc. The superficial glands may become enlarged and may suppurate.

In feeble constitutions the sufferings of the patients are variable, depending largely on the complications; it is, however, out of proportion to the skin lesions. Burning, followed by roughness, and a feeling of constriction may be present. It is a disease of adult life, occurring between the age of forty and sixty years, and is more common to men than to women. It may occur as a secondary manifestation in eczema, psoriasis, pemphigus.

Pathology—It is essentially an inflammation of the skin, involving principally the epidermic layers, but in the chronic forms the deeper layers of the corium become involved. Atrophy of the hair follicles with separation of the corneal layers of the epidermis.

Etiology—The etiology of this disease is obscure, as many cases occur apparently without previous ill health. The history of rheumatism is usually present although many authors believe it to be a trophoneurosis.

Diagnosis—The disease is apt to be confounded with erythema, scarlatiniforme, eczema rubrum, pemphigus, foliæus, psoriasis and lichen.

In eczema rubrum the eruption is more local, color lighter, itching and moisture always present. In dermatitis it is always dry and has no crusts, besides it is more rebellious to treatment.

Pemphigus is also a moist eruption, is accompanied with bullæ and a peculiar sickening odor. Only in exceptional and exaggerated cases should it be mistaken for psoriasis, but the adherent pearl colored scales heaped up or piled upon each other and adherent are quite unlike dermatitis.

In lichen rubrum and lichen planus the lymphatic glands are not involved, constitutional symptoms absent and the scales finer.

Treatment—The application of olive or sweet oils is soothing and modifies the sufferings of the patients; it is also a protection from cold and the atmosphere. The remedies most frequently called for are: Aco., Ars., Kali ars., Ars. iod., Piper. methy., Clem., Graph., Rhus, Sulph., Syphil., Tub., Psor., Lyc., Lach., Nat. mur., Sep.

DERMATITIS MEDICAMENTOSA (Drug Eruption)

DEFINITION—This form of dermatitis embraces all inflammatory processes due to the administration of drugs internally or externally.

SYMPTOMS—Dermatitis medicamentosa does not cover the whole field of dermatitis induced by drugs or local irritants, but simply those coming under general use in medicine. The continuation of the subject usually comes under the heading of dermatitis venenata, which includes any medicinal substance capable of producing inflammations of the skin, whether vegetable or mineral.

In our study of this subject we find every variety of lesion similar to those found in other diseased conditions, such as macules, papules, pustules, wheals, tubercles, vesicles, bullæ ulcerations, and even the most profound manifestations of sloughing and gangrene.

In some cases identical effects follow the application of drugs in the different patients we meet; again they may be quite dissimilar. The reason for this we may look for as in all other diseases, knowing that disease is a disturbance of the life force; hence the phenomena will depend much on what kind of a life force is disturbed, be it tubercular, sycotic, or psoric. Sometimes we find them confined to the point of local contact; again, similar lesions will appear in other parts; the local effects are, however, more constant, and the degree of which depends much on the susceptibility and sensitivity of the individual.

The eruptions appear within a few minutes to hours after the application or contact, developing rapidly and vanishing sooner or later after the removal of the exciting cause. The lesions may be single or multiple, and the most common anatomical seat is upon the exposed or unclothed parts, unless applied as local irritants, dressings, etc. Almost any sensation may be present upon the skin, such as itching, pricking, tingling, smarting, burning, even to pain itself; constitutional symptoms may or may not be present.

Etiology—Women and children suffer more than men, due to their greater sensitivity. Children are more apt to have reflex or constitutional symptoms. This, together with the peculiarity of diathesis, renders the difference of degree and intensity of the disease.

Pathology—The disease is due to nutritive or atrophic and reflex disturbances similar to those seen in urticaria.

INDICATIONS—*Boracic acid* produces a bluish erythema, with macules, pustules, urticaria and bullæ, together with scaly patches, similar to psoriasis.

Carbolic acid—Marked erythema, extending even beyond the affected surface, vesicles, pustules, even ulceration and gangrene.

Salicylic acid—Urticaria, vesicles, pustules, herpetic, pemphigoid, eruptions and petechia.

Aconite—Vesicular dermatitis, bullæ and erysipelatous inflammations.

Anacardium—The tincture, fluid extract, and more especially the oil of the cashew, is an intense irritant of the skin, producing edematous infiltration, erythema, papules, vesicles and bullæ. The erythema takes on the form of an erysipelatous inflammation, similar to Rhus tox., and each may be an antidote to the other.

Antifebrin—Antifebrin and all the coal tar preparations are dangerous drugs (see literature of 1896 and 1897), Sajous's Annual and Analytical Cyclopædia of Practical Medicine, p. 417, Vol. I). The skin symptoms are quite marked. It produces a cold, clammy perspiration, with more or less cyanosis, blueness of the skin, and a bright red scarlet rash is occasionally seen. Its action upon the

7

heat is readily seen upon the skin. It produces bluish papules and exanthema like measles.

Arnica—Arnica is frequently used locally in injuries. It produces an erythema and vesicular eruptions very similar to Rhus tox., and is attended with burning and intense itching, bullæ, erysipelatous inflammations, purpuric spots. A few cases are reported terminating fatally. Great soreness and tenderness accompany these severe cases.

Arsenicum—Almost any lesion can be found from the use of, or rather the abuse of, Arsenic locally, even to ulceration and gangrene. The frequent use of Arsenic in the industries, such as artificial flowers, cards, boxes, dyes, wall paper, causing numerous disturbances and many forms of eruptions upon the skin. Grayish or brownish discoloration is often found upon the face, neck and abdomen after prolonged use of the drug; the pigmentation accompanying the eruption is often long lasting. Thickening of the palms of the hands, knuckles and soles of the feet have also been observed. The skin in chronic poisoning has a pale, grayish, cachectic appearance, dry, scaly, unhealthy looking; burning in the local lesion is quite a constant symptom.

Belladonna—Bright red erythema or scarlatina, like rash, vesicular erysipelatous eruptions. Belladonna plasters have often produced a local, intense dermatitis with marked vesication and followed by constitutional symptoms, fever, delirium and even convulsions in sensitive women and children.

Bromium—Bromium and its compounds produce many skin lesions of a papular, pustular nature, more especially the bromide of patash given so liberally in nervous and mental diseases, until the mental powers are almost destroyed, and a peculiar idiotic expression is observed upon the faces of those using it. After sometime a peculiar eruption is found upon the face, neck, scalp, back and chest, and is known as "chronic acne."

Erythema, urticaria, papillary, hypertrophy, vesicles, bullæ, nodules, furuncles, and even anthrax appear after long use of the drug.

Cantharides—This drug produced an intense dermatitis complicated with vesicles and large blebs, containing a yellowish, watery fluid; ulceration and gangrene has often been observed upon the affected surface. Erythema of an erysipelatous nature with papules, pustules, and vesicles are constant lesions; irritation of the urinary tract, strangulation, and even complete suppression of urine are some of the constitutional symptoms.

Chloroform—Produces a blotchy, erythematous rash, and occasionally purpuric spots.

Ergot—Ergot produces a vesicular eruption with petechia, pustules, and furuncles, with green pus, dark swellings, even phlegmonous inflammations.

Mercury—Mercury produces erythema and vesicular eruptions, and occasionally an intense dermatitis with sloughing. It also has produced urticaria, herpes, purpura, furuncles, impetigo.

Iodine and its compounds—While producing the well known yellowish-brown stain upon the skin it also produces papulo-pustular and bullous eruptions as well as erythema, which is followed by desquamation.

Quinine—Many forms of eruptions are seen after the overuse of quinine; it produces erythema, vesicles, bullæ, exfoliation of the skin, purpura, urticaria, and a rash similar to scarlatina.

Diagnosis—A good knowledge of the toxic action of the drug makes the diagnosis easy. The limitation of the inflammation to the exposed surface and its prompt disappearance upon the cessation of the action of the exciting cause are marked differential signs.

Etiology—The sensitivity and susceptibility are always marked etiological considerations from drug poisoning. Some patients seem to have a peculiar vital resistance to the action of certain poisons, while, on the other hand, they are extremely susceptible to them. Changes in health and conditions of the system, as well as planetary influences, have been shown to have their influences upon the susceptibility of the patient.

Treatment—A thorough cleansing of the part and a removal of the local cause as far as possible are the first things to be considered. The physiological antidote has sometimes to be resorted to, but usually the higher potencies selected and prescribed upon the totality of the symptoms give more satisfactory results. Often the highest potency that can be procured of the toxic element will have to be given to remove its secondary or dynamic effects from the system.

DERMATITIS CALORICA

Dermatitis Calorica comprises the two forms induced by direct opposite causes from heat and from cold. The dermoid disturbances from heat are called dermatitis ambustionis, and those from cold, dermatitis congelationis. Either may produce erythema, vesicles, sloughing, ulcerations, even death of the part. Therefore the conditions met with are similar in their ultimate results in the changing and destruction of tissue, although caused by opposite extremes from the zero temperature point.

Dermatitis Ambustionis—SYNONYM—Burns and scalds.

DEFINITION—All inflammatory processes and changes induced by dry or moist heat.

SYMPTOMS—Shoemaker divides burns and scalds into three classes, which seems to be the best method of classification. They are erythematous, bullous and escharotic. We may also retain the older classification into first, second and third degrees.

Dermatitis of the first degree is of the erythematous variety, although occasionally a few small vesicles may be found upon the seat of the lesion. It is usually due to the exposure of the summer sun, or coming in contact with steam, a flame, ignited gases, heated solids or liquids. The local symptoms are more or less painful, burning, smarting, with a reddened and slightly swollen surface. The symptoms soon disappear, however, with more or less desquamation of the epidermis, the age, sex and location of the lesion having much to do with the suffering of the patient.

BULLOUS FORM—The bullous form is due to a more protracted contact with any of the above forms of heat; bullæ or even blebs, of almost any size or shape, develop in the lesion, depending on the extent of the infiltration. The pain and inflammation are usually intense, and the neighboring glands are often affected in sympathy. The serum contains fibrinogen, and is coagulable. In some cases the repair takes place by crusting, but generally by granulation and cicatrization should the corium be destroyed.

The escharotic form or the third degree, known as the escharotic, or gangrenous form, is the result of an intense heat, or a continuous exposure, causing death of the skin, and often of the deeper structures. The integument may be dry or moist, and of any color from white to black, frequently without sensation. Carbonization may have taken place in all the underlying tissues. The skin surrounding the wound is usually intensely swollen, and if pain be not present at the time it follows soon after, inducing great suffering. In a few days, however, the death-line in the tissues is manifest, and the eschar is thrown off gradually, and granulation takes place slowly, and healing takes place by fibrous connective tissue, which is quite destitute of nerves and bloodvessels and the usual organs of the skin. The cicatrices generally contract, producing marked deformity, depending, of course, much on the anatomical seat of the lesion and the muscles involved.

Constitutional symptoms are always quite severe in the second and third forms. The degree of shock depending on the sensitivity of the patient, and the extent of destruction in the tissues, together with fever, pain, suppuration, ulceration and sloughing contribute to the suffering of the patient.

As secondary complications the kidneys and bladder may become involved, ulceration of the bowels, cerebral infusion, pneumonia, or pleurisy follow: hæmorrhages may follow in the suppurating process, or the sloughing and exhausting suppuration bring about a fatal termination.

Pathology—Alteration in the blood vessels inducing contraction and slowing of the circulation in the part. Thrombus may form in any part of the body, giving rise to venous stasis, or congestion to any organ, causing secondary complications.

Diagnosis—Classification is always of importance as to whether it is a scald or burn. The smell of fire or burning flesh, and the destruction of the hairs are of diagnostic value, while carbonization may be present, rendering the diagnosis easy.

Prognosis—Always guarded in view of secondary complications. The strength of the patient, age, sex, location, and extent of surface involved together with the ability of the patient to resist shock.

Treatment—Probably no other class of patients have received greater benefit or have more fully realized the wonderful efficacy and virtue of Homœopathy than those afflicted with burns. The promptness with which the pain and suffering is relieved by the well indicated remedy is truly remarkable. Frequently has the author seen patients suffering from the first and second degree so relieved from the pain and suffering as to allow them to fall asleep within thirty or forty minutes after taking the remedy; especially is this so in children. It can only be done, however, with the higher potencies.

The treatment of burns may require both surgical and medical aid, depending, of course, on the degree; prompt antiseptic cleansing of the part is necessary, although too frequent bathing is not recommendable, as it aggravates many cases. Local application of carron oil, sweet, or olive oil is soothing, and assists in keeping out the air, which is very irritating in the early stages of burns. Sterilized gauze well saturated with some one of the oils mentioned is the best dressing, although oiled silk may be required in some cases on account of its non-adhesive qualities. All medical applications are to be avoided if possible, as they suppress the local symptoms so necessary in the selection of the remedy, which in the end gives better results, and with less danger of secondary complications arising. Even the shock is less marked when medical applications are left off, and the properly selected remedy given in the beginning. There is also less loss of tissue, and a healthy granulation takes place at once.

Experience has shown that it is better not to open the vesicles, or blebs, as they are the best protection from the air; however, should it become necessary for drainage purposes, puncture them at their most dependent point. Skin grafting is only necessary in rare cases where extensor surfaces are involved. Contraction and deformity can be so modified, if not entirely relieved by the homœopathic remedy, so as to leave operative measures almost entirely out of the question. Rest, position, proper bandaging, good nursing and a suitable diet are all necessary considerations.

REMEDIES—Most frequently indicated are Aco., Bell., Canth., Amm. c., Apis, Ars., Carbo veg., Lach., Caust., Rhus tox., Urtica urens, Ruta, Coff., Camph., Phos., Chin. off., Terebinth.

INDICATIONS—*Aconite.* Aconite more especially in children, frequently indicated in the beginning of the treatment, for the febrile and nervous symptoms.

Belladonna—High fever with a drowsy, sleepy condition of the patient, quick, rapid pulse, much thirst for small drinks of water. The part very red, hot, tender and sensitive to touch, and in some cases convulsions.

Arnica—Arnica is often indicated when the burn is accompanied with traumatism, and where there is much shock, great soreness in the affected part.

Arsenicum—In very severe cases, accompanied with great prostration and fear of death, thirst for frequent sips of cold water, nausea and vomiting after drinking.

Complications arise in internal organs with great loss of strength; locally, frequently, a gangrenous condition is met with, also extensive ulceration and sloughing, with great burning and smarting of the part.

Carbo veg—Bil. mot. temp. Great prostration and tendency to hæmorrhages; the wound looks dark and unhealthy; its discharges are offensive, carrion-like, tendency to collapse; parts remote from center of circulation are cold; blebs dark, even black; pulse slow, feeble, weak, with great desire for cool air or to be fanned; extreme cases of shock; great burning, or complete loss of sensation.

Cantharis—Cantháris is frequently indicated in burns of the first and secondary degree; dark red or bluish erythema with intense biting, smarting and burning; burning intense, unbearable; large, painful, straw-colored blebs soon make their appearance after the burn; symptoms greatly aggravated by water and open air; urine scanty with tenesmus of the bladder, and sometimes strangulation or complete suppression. The suffering of the patient compels him to move about. This remedy should not follow camphor.

Apis—Great edema of the part with much stinging and burning; part tense, dry, hot, or pale and edematous about the lesion; urine scanty, dark colored, with painful urging; no thirst; symptoms better in the cool air.

Urtica urens—Prickling, burning, stinging, itching; distressing, burning heat, with formication; raised red blotches, with fine stinging points, better by lying down and by gentle rubbing. In children with vesical irritation.

Veratrum vir—Skin cold, clammy, blue, shrivelled, often insensible, intense fever with marked vesication, tingling, itching, prickling; severe burns with cerebral symptoms.

Terebinth—Severe burns accompanied with hæmorrhages from internal organs, dark red erythema with petechiæ and ecchymotic spots; blood or albumen passes in the urine after severe burns, congestions to the viscera, intense burning and smarting of the skin.

Rhus tox—Dark blue erythema with intense burning, stinging, itching, and smarting; great soreness and lameness of the part; extreme physical restlessness, which is relieved by walking or change in position.

Carburetum sulph—Frequently indicated in severe burns or scalds, brownish vesicles on a red, swollen base, containing an opaque, yellowish fluid; discharge forms thick yellow crusts.

Coffea, Ignatia, Opium, Gels., Hyos., Stram., will be frequently called for to meet the nervous symptoms arising from the effects of shock, especially in women and children.

DERMATITIS CONGELATIONIS

SYNONYMS—Frost bite, pernio, chilblain.

DEFINITION—This form of dermatitis is a painful inflammation, usually of the fingers, hands, toes, feet, due to exposure to cold, and accompanied with any degree of the inflammatory process, such as tenderness, erythema, vesication, ulceration, sloughing, or gangrene.

VARIETIES—There are three degrees as found in the division of burns and scalds: 1st. The general erythema. 2nd. Vesication or blebs. 3rd. The destruction of tissue with scar.

SYMPTOMS—On the first appearance the skin is white, cold, wrinkled, and dead-like, with partial or complete loss of sensation. If the cold is prolonged vesication is induced, and frequently the blebs contain a bloody serum. This may develop into the third stage, with death and sloughing of the affected part. As soon as the cold is removed the color changes, a marked inflammatory process is set up, and a line of demarkation separates the frozen from the healthy tissue, which soon suppurates and sloughs out, the constitutional symptoms being in proportion to degree, extent, and location of the lesion. The sloughing is always accompanied with an offensive odor.

CHILBLAINS—Chilblains are simply an after action or a development from the effects of frost bites in many psoric people. Chilblains appear periodically at the appearance of cold weather, beginning as an erythema, accompanied with an intense burning, tingling and itching, and sometimes followed by vesication and ulceration. It may become hereditary in some families, and suppressing it by local applications, such as camphor and other strong local medicants, has developed many severe forms of chronic diseases.

The writer recalls two cases of chorea, three of migraine and one severe case of stomach trouble. In three of these cases the eruption was re-produced, after having been suppressed for years. I know of no condition, except it be sycosis, that, if suppressed, will develop more spasmodic or severely painful diseases than suppressed chilblains. There is probably a sycotic element at the bottom of chilblains.

Diagnosis—Symptoms are so characteristic as to allow no possible chance for error.

Prognosis—Prognosis of burns, if of the first degree, always favorable, but if of the second or third degree, surgical means may have to be employed. The probability of shock and general heart failure are not to be forgotten in our diagnosis.

Treatment—The treatment, as in burns, is both medicinal and surgical. The patient should be placed in bed in a cool room, if of the second or third degree, and the part affected bathed with ice water, snow or crushed ice, applied until the circulation is restored; then dress as in suppurating wounds.

The remedies as given under burns and scalds may be consulted, as well as any other of the antipsorics, as the constitutional symptoms are very similar under each. However, in the chronic condition known as chilblains, a consultation of the following remedies and some of their indications may be of some assistance to us:

REMEDIES—Abrot., Agar., Arn., Badiag., Cadm. sulph., Carbo veg., Rhus tox., Pet., Puls., Bell., Lyc., Tub., Phos., Zinc.

INDICATIONS—Agaricus. Acquired or hereditary chilblains, dark, purple or bright red blotches, with a marked periodicity of the appearance of the eruption. Electriclike shocks, pricking, as of needles, redness of the part, with intense burning, biting, stinging and itching; indicated in light-haired people with lax muscle.

Ammonium carb—Violent itching after rubbing, with burning vesicles following. At night the itching and stinging keeps him awake. Eruption dark blue, worse in the evening and during the new moon, also, in cold air; better by warmth and by bandaging.

Belladonna—Bright red, shiny swelling of the part, very sensitive to touch, tingling and itching, worse from touch.

Petroleum—Tubercular patients with moist chilblains, parts painfully swollen and red, pustules form, itch and burn like fire, chilly sensations throughout the body accompanying the itching. Chilblains of the hands, heels, toes, accompanied with moisture.

Pulsatilla—Bluish red chilblains with prickling, burning pains, worse in the afternoon and evening, better by the cool air blowing on them. Symptoms changeable, worse after menses and when getting warm.

Rhus tox—Dark colored blotches with itching, burning, stinging; worse before storms or when getting wet. Chilblains with muscular pains throughout the body; the suffering is relieved by motion and gentle rubbing. Burning, stinging, smarting, itching with fine vesicles appearing on a dark blue erythematous base.

Tuberculinum—Frequently indicated in light blondes with blue eyes; tall, slim, flat, narrow-chested people, who have a family history of tubercular affections; and whose symptoms are ever changing, who take cold easy; eruption dry and scaly, itching intolerable, followed by long-lasting burning and smarting; better by warm bathing. Obstinate chronic cases with tubercular history.

Sulphur—Indicated in deeply psoric patients with chronic dry skin. Skin rough, pimply, eruption very red, itching intolerable; worse at night and by warmth of bed. Itching is better by scratching and rubbing, but produces burning and smarting. Feet burn at night, and the patient has a desire to put them out of bed, or find a cool place for them.

Syphilinum—Short memoried, forgetful subjects, chilblains with latent syphilitic complications, brownish red or bluish eruption, covered with fine, white scales, with great itching and burning. The part too sore to scratch; the symptoms are all aggravated at night and by warmth, like mercury; also, worse during the change of weather.

Psorinum—Pale, emaciated, very psoric people, who worry and fret very much about their condition, who have unhealthy, inactive skin, and who do not perspire; they are extremely sensitive to cold, dirty, tawny colored eruption, with fine scales over the surface, disappearing during the warm weather, but reappearing during the cold; fingers and toes are so swollen they can't flex them, with desquamation of fine scales. Suppressed cases are often reproduced by this remedy. Local symptoms: intense itching, burning and biting, scratching until it bleeds.

LICHEN RUBER (Pityriasis Pilaris)

DEFINITION—It is characterized by an eruption of small, red acuminate papules about the orifices of the hair follicles, forming by aggregations large patches covered with fine, whitish scales; sometimes it involves the whole surface of the body. It has a tendency to run a slow, changeable course, and to verge into a chronic state.

SYMPTOMS—Prodromal symptoms are absent, the disease being announced by the sudden appearance of small, mustard-seed sized, conical-shaped, red or reddish brown papules, which, when fully developed, undergo no change. They are firm to touch, and have fine scales on their apex. The disease develops upon any portion of the body. It begins usually on the extremities; more or less itching is present. There are three forms mentioned by the authorities, the papular, squamous and rugous, but each depends on a more marked development or expression of the lesion.

In the rugous form the patches show marked depression in the natural furrows of the skin. The white scales having fallen off, leaving a dull, red, leathery hue. In chronic or relapsing cases the skin shows marked infiltration, forming dry, brittle, leathery, fissured, scaly patches, often causing the eyelids to droop, or, if upon the lips, they become thickened and indurated. The palms of the hands and soles of the feet also become thickened, hardened, and fissured, making motion painful, and causing much suffering. The hair and nails become brittle, and the former frequently falls out. The nails also may be cast off, generally being found ridged, thickened, and of a grayish color.

There are no constitutional symptoms except where the eruption extends over a large portion of the body, when the digestive and assimilative functions become seriously disturbed, the appetite fails; sleep is disturbed, and the patient gradually emaciates; a general marasmic condition may follow, or some inter-current disease cause a fatal result.

Diagnosis—Simple forms of the disease may be taken for acne, papular eczema, papular syphilide, lichen planus. The papules of acne are larger and occur on the face, and usually become pustular. In papular eczema the papules itch intensely and run an acute course, or change into some other lesion. In psoriasis the patches are smaller, more circular, and covered with thick, white, silvery scales which, when detached, bleed from pin-point surfaces. In syphilis the lesions become pustular, and are very apt to be copper colored, and have no subjective symptoms. The papules of lichen planus are larger in size than the ruber, showing a depressed or umbilicated appearance, disappear by resolution, leaving a pigmentation with atrophy of the epidermis, and the hairs are not affected.

Pathology—Marked hypertrophy of all the layers of the corium. The cells of the rete are completely changed, the papillæ increased in size, and the bloodvessels dilated. The disease is considered by many authors as an hyperkeratosis.

Etiology—The cause of lichen ruber is yet a mystery.

Treatment—For treatment consult psoriasis.

LICHEN PLANUS

DEFINITION—This is an inflammatory disease of the skin marked by an eruption of flattened, dull red, shiny papules, with a central depression, a tendency to coalesce, and to form into patches.

SYMPTOMS—The lesions are at first discrete, but show a marked tendency to aggregate into irregular patches of various sized lines or circles. They never pustulate or vesicate. The eruption appears first upon the anterior surfaces, forearms, legs, and trunk. It pursues a chronic course, and disappears by resolution, leaving a pigmented, rough, and uneven surface.

Pathology—The microscope shows a mass of round cells in the papillary layer of the corium, with thickening of the rete. The papules are formed usually around the sweat ducts, which give rise to the umbilicated appearance.

Etiology—The disease is rare in children, usually beginning between the thirtieth and fortieth year of adult life. It occurs in those patients suffering from mental or nervous diseases having a rheumatic or gouty tendency, suggesting the manifestation of some form of sycosis.

Treatment—The nourishment of the patient is important, together with the careful selection of the homœopathic remedy. The diet should consist of vegetables, cereals, eggs, milk, etc.

The remedies to be considered are: Ant. cru., Arn., Ars., Agar., China, Ars. iod., Sep., Kali iod., Sarsap., Led., Cal. c., Dul., Lyc., Nux jug., Puls., Phos., Phos. ac., Merc.

PART III

CLASSIFICATION—DISEASES OF SECRETION AND EXCRETION

DISEASES OF THE SWEAT GLANDS

DEFINITION.—A functional disorder of the sweat glands characterized by increased or abnormal sweating.

FORMS.—There are four special forms, hyperidrosis, anidrosis, bromidrosis, chromidrosis.

HYPERIDROSIS

DEFINITION—An excessive secretion of perspiration due to a functional disturbance of the sweat glands.

Symptomatology—It may be partial or general, acute or chronic. A profuse general sweating may occur in comparatively healthy individuals, especially in the nervous or the lymphatic, after violent exercise or the ingestion of large quantities of fluids, or from any marked increase of temperature. It may be considered unnatural, however, in the absence of those natural conditions. When the disease presents itself locally it is met with more frequently on the face, hands, feet, genitals, which is usually due to faulty innervation. It may be due to diseased conditions of the brain or spinal centers. The diseases of the brain often produce excessive sweating; acute diseases, exophthalmic goitre, delirium tremens, lead poisoning, diseases of the kidneys, hysteria, and other nervous diseases.

Diagnosis—The diagnosis is never difficult.

Etiology—The miasm psora and latent syphilis is

usually clearly manifest in these patients, and the disease should never be suppressed, either by local medication, medicated baths, or any other local means whatever, as you are simply closing up the sewer gates of the body; for through the medium of perspiration the whole organism is more simply and effectively relieved of the miasmatic poisons than through any other eliminative process of the body.

Treatment—The treatment should consist of frequent bathing with warm or tepid water, together with a careful selection of the homœopathic remedy, which should be based upon the miasmatic symptoms of the patient. Shields and other such protection may be used temporarily until such times as the selected remedy will have removed the cause entirely from the system.

ANIDROSIS

DEFINITION—Decreased or diminished perspiration due to some disturbance of the sweat glands.

Symptomatology—The disease may be idiopathic or symptomatic, general or local, congenital or hereditary. In some people we find an increased secretion of the perspiratory fluid; in others it is greatly diminished, even absent, that is, the sensible perspiration. Ichthyosis is a typical example of an idiopathic case. The symptomatic form is more common, and may be local or general. It is generally met with in syphilis or tubercular patients. It is usually local, and quite often offensive, and excoriating in its nature, producing itching, burning and many other sensations, depending on the character of the secretion.

BROMIDROSIS

DEFINITION—Offensive perspiration.

Symptomatology—It also may be general or local,

usually local, occurring in the axilla, flexures of the body, genital regions, groins, hands and feet. The secretion may assume almost any odor, such as decayed cheese, onions, violets. Again it may be musty, sour, sweet, ammoniacal or carrion-like. The disease is usually more marked in summer than in winter.

Axillary, genital or foot sweats are found more frequently in tubercular or latent syphilitic patients. A suppressed foot sweat has often resulted in stasis to the lungs or other organs. Any condition, however, may arise from such suppressions, as neuralgia, headaches, vertigoes and other almost innumerable diseases, often only relieved or cured when the foot sweat is re-established.

The secondary local symptoms that may arise are itching, smarting, rawness, soreness, etc., of the part. Frequently the epidermis looks white, as if scalded, wrinkled or red and excoriated.

CHROMIDROSIS

DEFINITION—Colored sweat.

Symptomatology—This disease is also called a functional disorder, but the homœopathic physician, who sees deeper into the mysteries of the disturbed life force, recognizes it as one of nature's eliminative processes, depending on one or more of the chronic miasms. It is a rare disease, however, and the perspiration may be increased or decreased in quantity, and of almost any color; yellowish, greenish, reddish, bluish, brown or even black; or, in fact, any modification of these colors. It is never constant, but comes and goes.

The disease is met with more frequently in women who suffer with uterine or nervous disorders, and more frequently on the face, chest, arms, hands and feet.

Treatment—Baryt. car., Bry., Ars., Cal. c., China, Con., Crocus, Ferr., Jabor., Kali c., Phos., Phos. ac., Acetic ac., Samb., Selen., Sep., Sil., Thuja, Mer. c., Mur. ac., Carb. veg., Iod., Psor., Sulph., Hepa, Picrotoxine, Pilocarp., Laur., Lach., Stan., Lyc., Pet., Baryt. mur., Baryt. iod., Nit. ac., Syph., Ant. cr., Medorrh., Nat. mur., Sabad., Staph.

INDICATIONS—*Calc. carb.*—Sang. Lymph. temp. Location, face, scalp, forehead and upper part of body; profuse perspiration occurring in infants and children, coming out in large colorless beads, while asleep or when nursing, which is frequently a sign that the child is not assimilating the bone-making constituents from its food. Tubercular children with large heads and open sutures, and with soft, flabby muscles.

China off—Bil. mot. temp. Profuse, general, exhausting, colorless and odorless perspiration, after acute or chronic exhausting diseases; ceases when awake and when moving about, but returns when asleep; great exhaustion after sweating.

Lycopodium—Sang. mot. temp. Profuse sweating, more about the face, scalp and upper part of the body. Worse in the evening. Profuse sour smelling, offensive, even bloody; much thirst after sweating.

Arsenicum—Sang. vit. ment. temp. Sweats during sleep, the entire night, cold, clammy, folowed by much prostration, occasionally offensive, cold perspiration on different parts of the body, better after sleep, shuddering when uncovered.

Baryta carb—Sang. lymph. temp. Effective foot and axillary sweat, left-sided sweating, sweating with anxiousness, which is increased in the presence of strangers and by eating; indicated in the sang. lymp. temp., or in fat people who suffer from glandular enlargement, or diseases of children; in the first and second childhood; offensive foot sweat, where the toes and soles of the feet become raw, and excoriated from the perspiration.

Kali carb—Bil. vit. temp. Profuse, warm sweat that does not relieve. Sweat of tubercular patients that is worse from least exertion and after midnight, profuse night sweats with a dry tubercular cough (Tub.).

Lachesis—Bil. nervo. lymph. temp. Profuse, strong, garlic-smelling axillary sweat. The sweat stains the linen brown or yellow. The odor is carrion-like (Psor.). Worse during sleep, in typhoid and exhausting fevers. Climacteric sweating following flushes of heat (Sulph.).

Nat. mur—A profuse sweat, with thirst, which relieves all the symptoms (reverse Mer.). The skin is yellowish, dry or dirty looking, perspiration causes soreness and intertrigo. Vesicles and herpes; worse from ten o'clock to three. Perspiration often tastes salty.

Mercurius—Sang. ment. vit. temp. Perspires very easily from the least exertion, worse drinking warm drinks, worse at night when asleep; profuse, offensive, sour, debilitating, wrinkling the skin, or perspiration of the face, while the rest of the body is dry, cold, oily, clammy, greasy; staining the linen yellow. All the complaints are aggravated by sweating. Tongue pasty, thickly coated, showing the imprints of the teeth; taste insipid or metallic.

Jaborandi—Copious sweating with salivation; perspiration starts from the forehead and face and spreads all over the body.

Silicea.—Sang. ment. mot. temp. Sweat of the head, face, feet, hands, and axilla (Cal. c.). Offensive foot sweat, carrion-like odor, scalding the part, producing soreness and rawness; profuse perspiration of the child's head, wetting the pillow, worse during sleep (Calc.);

9

sour, offensive, debilitating; worse after midnight; phthisis; hands and feet always cold and clammy (Calc. c.); patient canont bear to be uncovered; takes cold easily; indicated in chilly, pale-skinned, light-complected, latent syphilitic, or tubercular patients.

Iodine—Bil. mot. temp. Dark-complected, irritable people, who are subject to glandular enlargements; profuse, cold, debilitating, viscid perspiration, staining the linen yellow, and accompanied with rapid emaciation. The skin is dry, rough, dirty yellow; offensive sweat of the feet, hands, and axilla, axillary sweat rots the linen or shields (Sep., Sil., Psor.).

Thuja—Sang. lymph. temp. Sweats on covered parts during sleep; oily, fetid, or sweetish-smelling foot-sweats in sycotic patients after gonorrhea; biting in the skin as of insects after perspiration.

Sulphur—Sang. mot. ment. temp. Copious, sour, early morning sweat all over the body. The sweat has a burnt odor, skin dry, hot, burning in the early part of the night, with great restlessness.

Syphilinum—Excessive, general debilitating night-sweats, more marked between the scapula and around the waist; sleepless and restless; disagreeable musty odor of perspiration.

Staph—Bil. vit. temp. Perspiration smells like rotten eggs, with desire to uncover during perspiration.

Sepia—Bil. mot. temp. Sweat from nervous shock or other causes; worse on the back, chest, and flexures of the body; sour or offensive, or smelling like elder blossoms; foot-sweat causes soreness of the toes (Sil., Iod., Baryt. c.). Sweat colors the linen brown (Iod., Nit. a.); very difficult to wash out; indicated in women with nervous disorders and uterine troubles.

ACNE

DEFINITION—Acne is an inflammatory disease of the *sebaceous* glands of the skin and hair follicles, characterized by the presence on the face usually of small papules or nodules varying in size from a pin-head to a pea; this is of course the simple form; they appear on the face, nose, cheeks, chin, neck, shoulders, back.

SYMPTOMS—The lesions are solid, conical-shaped elevations, somewhat painful to pressure; there is a marked tendency to a suppurative change. In the centre of the papule a yellowish-white spot forms where the pus raises the epidermis. In from three to ten days they break open and a small amount of pus is discharged.

At other times the discharge dries into a thin crust, or the contents are absorbed together with the lesion; the surrounding skin has, as a rule, a greasy, oily appearance. Tumors from the size of a large pea to that of a hazel nut are sometimes met with, which often remain in a stationary condition for months, then disappearing or forming hard spherical indurations by retraction and inspissation of their contents. Scarring usually consisting of a small, white cicatricial depression is to be seen as a result in some cases. Permanent pitting or scarring is not a constant symptom by any means.

VARIETIES—There are several varieties of acne observed, one form of which is apt to predominate.

Acne vulgaris or acne simplex is by far the most common we meet with clinically; the lesions are of a multiple or mixed character and appearing as pin-head or pea-sized papules, papulo-pustules, and pustules. Sometimes these little papules may, when first seen, show a small, minute, transparent vesicle on their tops, which later on changes to a pustule, and finally disappears by the suppurative process.

Acne papulosum is that form which appears as papules and remains a papule throughout, showing very little tendency to suppurate, retaining the normal color of the skin, except in some cases a reddish areola may surround them in the earlier stages. They disappear by absorption or by dessication and exfoliation.

Acne punctata is a very minute papular lesion with a central comedo or black head, the discoloration being due to excrementitious matter.

Acne Pustulosum—This type goes rapidly into a pustule or into the pustular stage; in size they do not vary from the other varieties; the pus may be of a yellowish or even bloody color, usually thick and often of a cheesy consistency; sometimes they are quite sore and painful; crusting is usually present in some degree in this form; many of the papules, however, do not go beyond the primary lesion; they are more apt to be found in the strumous diathesis, the tubercular and the sycotic or gouty; of course, there can be no positive rule applied, as frequently we find the disease more prevalent in neurotic patients who are extremely psoric. No subjective symptoms are present to speak of except it be slight soreness, tenderness and some itching and burning.

Acne Indurata—This form may be safely said to depend wholly on a tubercular taint or diathesis as a basis. The lesions are deep seated, from the size of a pea to that of a small nut; not only are the sebaceous glands themselves affected, but the surrounding tissues are inflamed, hardened and indurated; enlarged, red or purplish in color, running an indolent course, requiring weeks sometimes to soften. They are round or irregular in shape, indolent, as a rule, in their progressive changes; sometimes they break down into small abscesses, but usually a very small amount of pus is discharged. The lesions slowly undergo resolution, are quite often painful to touch or pressure, and show, as a rule, marked scarring, and the lesion remains livid or purplish for a long space of time, having a tendency to run a chronic course with periods of outbreaks and apparent recovery. They appear on the face, neck, shoulders, nose, chin, back; often they will be found only on the back, and are aggravated at some phase of the moon, and if the patient be a woman, at the menstrual period. The general health may or may not be disturbed. They do not, however, as a rule, disappear spontaneously after the twenty-fift year, or about that time, as do the simple forms.

Artificial forms of acne are quite common in neurotic patients, due to the ingestion of such drugs as the iodides and bromides; also, by the external applications of certain local drugs, as tar, paraffin, oils, etc.

Etiology—Acne begins usually near puberty, when the whole glandular system of the skin is actively developing and their functions increasing. The fact that these patients suffer from constipation, dilation of the stomach, digestive troubles, menstrual irregularities, gouty conditions as well as neurotic troubles, is no proof that any of the above-mentioned diseases are the cause of this disease; rather are they developments and manifestations from the same underlying diathesis that causes the acne in the first place. Uterine irritation and disturbances of the digestive tract, diet, especially rich foods, meats, coffee, shell fish, beer. wines, spirituous liquors, are the most common of the secondary causes for careful consideration in the treatment of these many, difficult and stubborn forms of acne.

Pathology—In most cases the disease begins as a perifolliculitis, the sebaceous gland itself is the starting point of the inflammatory process, limited often to the sebaceous or pilary canal. If the inflammatory process is very great the gland may be entirely destroyed. The process may be divided into two parts, the closure of the sebaceous follicle and formation of comedo; second, the suppurative process.

Diagnosis—It may resemble syphilis in the papillary form, but in syphilis usually the history of the case, the color of the skin, and the suddenness of the invasion make the diagnosis not at all difficult.

Treatment.—The general health of the patient above everything is to be consulted in the treatment of this disease as far as therapeutic measures are concerned. One thing certain, you cannot treat the acne as a disease as it is only an expression of some internal disturbance we must necessarily correct, and in proportion as we correct it the acne will disappear. The deepest acting antimiasmatics will have to be studied in these chronic cases, as they are all dependent on a deep-seated constitutional and generally hereditary taint. Above all things, in taking these cases it is important to give yourself plenty of time, as the patient is very apt to make light of the case, there being no special constitutional symptoms to deal with present. Many cases will require a nourishing diet, while others will have to be deprived of such articles of food as fats, meats; pork above all other articles of food is to be condemned as an article of diet. Coffee, spices of all kinds are to be prohibited, as well as wines, beers and stimulants of all kinds; fresh air; walking as an exercise, together with a careful regulation of the habits, will aid materially in the cure of these cases. Cool, tepid baths, rubbing of the skin to increase the local circulation, will sometimes be of benefit.

Remedies—Acne vulgaris. Ars., Bell., Asaf., Alum., Cal. ☿., Cal. phos., Carbo veg., Dig., Dros., Graph., Grat., Carbol., Caust., Can. sat., Nat. mur., Nat. sulph., Nat. c., Nit. ac., Nux vom., Nux jug., Sabad., Sulph., Sabina, Selen., Sil., Sep., Hep., Sulph., Led., Baryta carb., Lach., Phos., Puls., Agar., Ant. crud, Ant. tart., Tub., Psor. Syph., Medorrh., Iod., Brom., Kali c., Kali iod., Bry., Dulc., Rhus, Sars., Staph., Lyc., Rheum, Plat., Bov., Pet., Mer. viv., Mer. sol., Mer. cor., Iod., Mag. carb.

Acne indurata. Calc. c., Carbo veg., Led., Sulph., Tab., Psor., Medorrh., Syph., Hep., Sulph. iod., Iod., Kali brom., Kali iod., Ars., Sil., Fluor. acid, Sep., Am. carb., Graph., Nat. mur.

Acne punctata (black points). Sulph., Nat. mur., Cal. c., Ars., Dios., Graph., Sabin., Aur., Bry., Dig., Eugenia, Plumb., Selen., Thuja, Tub., Mer. viv.

Acne rosacea. Carb. an., Carbo veg., Ars., Kreosot., Mez., Rhus, Ruta, Verat. alb., Cal. c., Cann. ind., Cicut., Kali iod., Led., Nit. ac., Phos., Sil., Thuja, Alum., Aur. mur., Caps., Nux v., Clem., Lach., Petr., Sulph., Sulph. ac., Sep.

PART IV

CLASSIFICATION—HYPERTROPHIES

CHLOASMA

DEFINITION—Chloasma is a pigmentary disease of the skin, attended by partial or general discoloration of the skin.

Symptomatology—It appears in one or more smooth patches, and the color is usually light brown or black, and due either to idiopathic or symptomatic causes. The former to external causes, as injuries, wounds, blows, pressure, friction or to diseased conditions, as eczema, or to local applications upon the skin. The symptomatic form is due to reflex or systemic diseases, such as syphilis, cancer, uterine affections, pregnancy, etc. The spots occur more frequently upon the face, hands or upon the trunk.

Pathology—The pigmentary deposit is in the rete-mucosum.

Etiology—The etiology has already been given in the symptomatology.

Treatment—The treatment consists in the removal of the local causes, if any, and directing the treatment to the constitutional symptoms of the patient.

NAEVUS PIGMENTOSUS

DEFINITION—Naevus is a pigmentary disease. It may be congenital or acquired. It consists in hypertrophy of the connective tissue, together with pigmentary deposit in excess. They are all dimensions, and may be round, oval or irregular. They vary in color from yellow to black, and may be elevated, or on a level with the skin. They are smooth, rough or uneven, single or multiple, and appear on any part of the body, but more frequently upon the face, head and neck. They are usually light or dark red in color, occasionally following the course of nerve tracks; their growth is generally slow, and may or may not disappear on pressure.

Pathology—Excessive pigmentary deposit, with excessive connective tissue hypertrophy.

Etiology—They are of sycotic origin.

Prognosis—They are usually permanent and difficult to remove by treatment.

CALLOSITIES

Definition—Callosities are hypertrophies of the horny layer of the epidermis, consisting of patches of thickened epidermis of a grayish or yellowish brown color.

Symptomatology—The surface of the skin is thick, firm, dense, generally smooth, but when large surfaces are involved it is rough and furrowed.

They are circumscribed; in size, from a five cent piece to that of the whole plantar surface. They are gradual in their development, occurring on the plantar or palmar surfaces. Sometimes they are complicated with inflammation, which has a tendency to remove them.

Pathology—Simple hypertrophy, with excessive epithelial growth.

Etiology—They may occur in the various trades and occupations of life, and are due to some form of pressure or mechanical irritation.

Treatment—Treatment may be both surgical and medicinal.

CLAVIS (Corns)

Definition—Corns are circumscribed hypertrophies of the epidermis, occurring more frequently about the small joints of the extremities.

Symptomatology—There are two varieties, the soft and the hard corn. The soft usually occurs between the toes, where there is more or less moisture from the coopted surfaces. The hard corns appear on more exposed surfaces.

A corn differs from a callosity in that it has a prig or pivot of pressure, and is found on the under-surface of the epithelium, which produces pain on pressure. They are more circumscribed than a callosity. They may be single or multiple, of the natural color of the skin, but occasionally they are of a yellowish-white color. The pain and sensitiveness is greatly aggravated in wet and stormy weather.

Pathology—Simple hypertrophy of the horny layer of the epidermis.

Etiology—They are due, no doubt, to mechanical pressure, yet every person does not have corns, so that we have no hesitancy in saying the diathesis, as a predisposing cause, lies behind their appearance. They are found more frequently in the latent syphilitic and those having a tubercular taint. These patients, of course, are all sensitive to barometric changes, hence the aggravation.

Treatment—Innumerable are the palliative means and methods that are employed in relieving these patients suffering from corns, yet in the end they are only palliative. The carefully selected constitutional remedy will do more to relieve the patient permanently than all other means combined.

Remedies—Ant. crud., Arn., Bry., Rhus tox., Sep.,

Bell. per., Sil., Pet., Lyc., Nit. ac., Sulph., Borax, Caust., Nat. mur., Nat. phos., Mag. aust., Graph., Fluor. ac., Thuja, Cal. c., etc.

VERRUGA

SYNONYM—Warts.

DEFINITION—Warts are little papilomatous growths of sycotic origin, covered with a hypertrophied layer of the epidermis.

Symptomatology—Verrucas are classified under different forms, which is, in a clinical way, valuable, as it designates the type of growth. They are Verruca Vulgaris, Verruca Plana, Digitata, Filiformis, and Acuminata.

VERRUCA VULGARIS

Verruca Vulgaris may be hereditary or acquired. They occur, however, more frequently in children after the first dentition. They may be moist or dry, single or multiple; they appear from the size of a pin-head to that of a pea, and even larger. They are firm, rugous, sessile, conical, or flat. They are largely limited to the hands; may be found, however, in other parts of the body. They vary in color from the normal skin to a yellowish, brownish, and even black. The deeper the color, usually, the longer has been the development. Excrementitious matter has much to do with the coloring or shading of this form. They are seldom painful or sensitive to touch.

Verruca Plana—The form of this variety is flat, broad, generally round in form, and size from that of a split pea to that of a ten cent piece; grayish, yellowish, or brownish in color, smooth or slightly roughened, single or multiple. They appear on the face, hands, trunk, in middle-aged people. They may be separated or grouped together. They cannot be said to be a true wart.

Verruca Digitata—This form is frequently met with on the scalp, back, or shoulders. They are finger-like, lobulated growths, flat, broad, with a carb-like appearance, whitish, reddish, or yellowish in color, occurring more frequently in women than in men, and at adult life.

Verruca Acuminata—This form, sometimes called the pointed condyloma or moist fig-pointed wart, is a true venereal growth, yet it is no more venereal than the other forms in the sense of being venereal, except that they partake of two venereal diseases instead of one, syphilis and sycosis combined. They occur upon the genital organs or about the mucous orifices of the body, along the borders of the mucous surface of the skin. They may be single or multiple, of a pinkish or dark red color, dry or moist, but they are usually found secreting a puriform, yellowish-green secretion of a very offensive odor. In form they may be club-shaped, cauliflower, cock's comb, or mulberry-shaped.

Pathology—They differ in the different varieties pathologically, yet they all have a connective tissue base from which springs a papillary excrescence. In the condylomatous form the papilla are greatly hypertrophied, but the horny layer absent. When the secretion is removed from them they appear vividly red, bleed easily on being irritated, although not very sensitive to touch. They are found from the size of a cherry to that of a small egg.

Etiology—When we come to the etiology of verruca the homœopathic physician must take a wide departure from the general pathologist. For no one can follow the teachings of Hahnemann, or study closely the history and developments of gonorrhea without seeing the true relationship between it and all forms of verruca, except it be the acuminata form, which can only be produced by the joint effort of the two miasms, syphilis and sycosis. The vulgaris and filiformic forms of verruca stand out pathognomonically as a positive sign of either hereditary or acquired sycosis, due to gonorrheal infection. They cannot exist without the sycotic taint. In the hereditary sycotic child they make their appearance usually about the completion of the eruption of the temporary teeth, and in the acquired, at the close of the secondary or the beginning of the tertiary stage of gonorrheal sycosis, usually no sooner than the one hundredth day after infection. They are, together with the red mole, the first tertiary manifestation upon the skin. Their appearance is always favorable to the patient, more especially where some inflammatory process is going on in the genito-urinary tract, or where neuralgia, rheumatism, or gouty conditions are present.

The homœopathic remedy, in its reactive or curative process, often establishes an eruption of warts about the sexual organs, or upon the skin, either of the vulgaric or filiform variety. In the treatment of deep chronic diseases of internal organs, or in malignancies of any form, their appearance upon the skin is a good omen, and is frequently followed by a cure of the chronic condition. The experience of the author is, that where warts are suppressed either by excising, by cautery, mental healing, or charms, some internal condition of a gouty or other nature is certain to develop. Such diseases as gout, neuralgia, rheumatism, interstitial changes of the kidneys, or fibrous changes in any organ, stomach troubles, especially diseases of the pyloris, in fact, any condition may be set up due to suppression of any manifestation of sycosis.

9

Treatment—It is especially desirable, says a prominent author of diseases of the skin, "to give remedies that will have a tonic action upon the system, such as iron, cod-liver oil, arsenic, strychnine, etc.," a trial, in place of resorting at once to surgical measures, to remove the growth; and naturally enough they might be led to do so, seeing that many of the children of sycotic parents are often weak, anæmic and unhealthy looking, showing marked features of the workings of the sycotic dyscrasia. But great as the learning of the modern pathologists may be, who so clearly follow the toxic, as well as the dynamic action of syphilis and tuberculosis, in all its intricate and mysterious changes and alterations in the organism, they cannot see similar changes and processes of development in the most profoundly affected sycotic patients, whose sufferings are far more severe and whose death processes are more numerous.

Remedies—Some of the more important remedies are: Alum., Ant. c., Nit. ac., Argent. met., Ars., Baryt. c., Caust., Cham., Dulc, Lach., Kalm., Lyc., Mer., Iod., Ruta, Kali c., Nat. sul., Nat. carb., Nat. mur., Rhus tox., Phytol., Thuja, Cal. c., Cal. phos., Sep., Sil., Sulph., Medorrh., Psor., Staph., Tub., Sycot., Teucr., Mag. aust.

REPERTORY

Inflamed Warts—Am. carb., Bell., Ars., Caust., Nit. ac., Sep., Sil., Sulph., Thuja, Bov., Cal. c., Nat. carb., Lyc., Rhus tox., Ruta.

Warts with shooting pains.—Bov., Ars., Nit. ac.

Warts with sticking pains.—Bov., Nit. ac., Hep.

Stinging, sticking pains—Am. carb., Ant. crud., Bar. c., Calc. c., Caust, Hep., Lyc., Nit. ac., Sep., Sil., Staph., Thuja, Sulph.

Warts bleeding—Thuja, Nit. ac., Cal. c., Caust., Cinnab., Ferr., Lyc., Nat. c., Pho. ac., Rhus tox,, Staph., Kali c., Iod., Sycot., mer. sol.

Warts jagged.—Cal. c., Caust., Lyc., Nit. ac., Staph., Sabina, Thuja.

Warts pedunculated.—Caust., Dulc., Lyc., Medorrh., Thuja, Nat. mur., Sulph., Nat. s., Sabina, Sep., Sil., Sycot.

Warts smelling like old cheese.—Medorrh., Thuja, Nit. ac., Con., Hep., Nat. sulph.

Warts cauliflower-shaped.—Kali iod., Nit. ac., Staph., Medorrh., Mer. protoiod., Mer. iod. flav., Cinnab., Thuja, Sars., Lyc., Aur., Ars., Iod., Syph.

Warts large.—Caust., Dulc., Kali c., Nat. c., Nit. ac., Thuja, Sep., Medorrh.

Warts ulcerated.—Ars., Nat. c., Calc., Caust., Hep., Phos., Sil., Thuja, Mer. sol.

Warts seedy.—Calc., Caust., Medorrh., Nat. mur., Sep., Thuja, Bar. c., Berb., Con., Dulc., Fluor. ac., Lach., Psor., Sars., Sulph.

Warts smooth.—Ant. cr., Dulc., Psor., Ruta, Sulph.

Warts throbbing.—Cal. c., Kali c., Lyc., Petrol., Sep., Hep., Sil., Sulph., Merc. sol.

Warts, location, anus.—Aur., Benz. ac., Lyc., Mer. v., Nit. ac., Sep., Staph., Kali iod., Sil., Thuja, Syph., Medorrh.

Warts, location, sexual organs.—Mer. v., Medorrh., Thuja, Cinnab., Sycot., Staph., Benz. ac.

Warts, location, eyelids.—Berb., Cinnab., Nit. ac., Thuja.

Warts, location, face.—Caust., Dulc., Kali c., Sep., Phos. ac., Caust.

Warts, location, trunk.—Thuja, Nit. ac., Calc., Lyc., Sep., Sulph., Medorrh., Sabina, Sanic., Kali mur.

Warts, lower extremities.—Thuja, Camph., Sulph., Sep., Tub., Sycot., Cale.

Warts, location, hands.—Caust., Calc., Thuja, Nit. ac., Berb., Sulph., Sep., Bufo.

Warts, location, nose.—Caust., Thuja, Nit. ac.

Warts, location, cheek.—Sep., Caust., Calc., Thuja.

Warts, location, back.—Caust., Nat. carb., Thuja.

Warts, location, chest.—Nit. ac., Thuja, Medorrh., Calc.

Warts, location, feet.—Thuja, Calc., Sulph.

Warts, location, toes.—Thuja, Caust., Spig.

Warts, location, lips.—Caust., Con., Nat. mur., Nit. ac., Thuja.

ICHTHYOSIS

SYNONYM—Fish skin.

DEFINITION—Ichthyosis is a hereditary or congenital disease of the skin of hypertrophied nature, characterized by scaling off of the epidermis, dryness, roughness, and sometimes warty growths.

Symptomatology—There are three clinical types or forms, xerosis, ichthyosis simplex, and ichthyosis hystrix.

The xerosis, or xeroderma, is the common form, although the symptoms are less marked. It is milder and does not change much throughout life. The skin has an unwashed, dry, roughened appearance, lacking that oily appearance it usually has. Closely adherent, fine, whitish, or grayish-white scales form upon the surface of covered parts, more especially the anterior or extensor surfaces of the body. They are decidedly prominent, resembling keratosis pilaris. The disease is very mild during the warm summer months, almost disappearing, but to be renewed again in winter with all its former severity. It is generally more marked in middle life.

The simplex form comes earlier in life, soon after birth. The scales are larger and the surface of the skin is marked by polyhedral interspaces similar to a tiled floor. The color of the scales is from a dull white to a dark red color; like the former disease, it is more marked in cold climates, especially in winter. There is almost no perspiration, therefore the body presents that dry, harsh, roughened, scaly appearance similar to the scales of a fish. The hair is also dry and lustreless. If the scales are forcibly removed, or even between the scales, the form of the blood-vessels can be seen. Itching, soreness, tenderness, and many very annoying or abnormal sensations are present during the cold season of the year. Yet these patients do not complain much from cold, nor do they suffer much from heat.

Ichthyosis Hystrix—This form manifests itself in the usual phenomena of the other forms, although the disease is not so general over the body. There are often seen zones of healthy skin, the face being seldom affected, and the affected part circumscribed. Often the severest manifestations of the disease are seen upon the palms of the hands and the soles of the feet, the whole surface having a thickened, leathery appearance, covered with dense horny caps, varying in size from that of a pea to that of a large tumor of a reddish brown, dark green, or even blackish color. Sometimes these growths are elevated several centimeters above the surface of the normal skin; should these caps be forcibly removed, a slightly bleeding surface with hypertrophied papillæ is seen beneath. The disease may remain stationary for a long time, or it may disappear spontaneously without any apparent reason. It sometimes disappears as the result of other diseases. Occasionally exfoliation of these horny plates takes place, only to reform again.

Pathology—Like most forms of skin hypertrophy there is seen a true hypertrophy of the epidermis and papillary layer of the corium.

Etiology—The disease, being congenital, is of course directly or indirectly inherited, often, however, passing over several generations. It has frequently been noticed to follow up one side of the family, that is, only the boys were affected, and *vice versa* the girls. This, we know, is peculiar to alopecian syphilis, as well as other diseases of syphilis, also of psoriasis.

Diagnosis—The early appearance of the disease, soon after birth, the rough, dry, scaly, polygonal plates, dirty gray in color, together with that general appearance of the skin of a fish, renders the diagnosis easy.

Prognosis—Not very favorable, years of treatment being required to cure these subjects.

Treatment—Change of climate does much for these patients, high, dry mountain air, or a prolonged sea voyage greatly relieves them; but it is prone to return, sooner or later, until the constitutional dyscrasia is rectified. Warm bran water baths are soothing. The free use of olive oil relieves the dryness to some extent, modifies the irritation and softens the skin in a mechanical way, as there are no natural secretions.

REMEDIES—The remedies from which we have seen the best results in this disease are: Ars, Ars. iod., Syph., Tub., Psor., Sulph., Graph., Aur., Cal. c., Mer. sol., Nuph. lutea, Pet., Phos., Sarracen, Tell., Teucr., Sep., Hydrocotyle, Iod., Lyc., Sil.

Arsenicum alb., Ars. iod., Syph., Psor., Tub., Petrol., Graph. have done more in my hands in the curing of this disease than all other remedies.

PSORIASIS

DEFINITION—Psoriasis is a non-contagious, cutaneous disease, characterized by the appearance of silvery white, or pearly-colored, dry scales, which overlie a reddish, shining base.

SYMPTOMS—It begins with small pin-head, rose-colored spots, that increase in size from the periphery. In a day or two following their appearance, and without any premonitory symptoms, they become covered with white silvery scales. If these be removed a reddish, slightly bleeding surface appears. These small, scaly lesions appear more frequently in children and are called punctate. When they increase in size they are called guttate, and when they assume the size of silver coins they are described as nummular psoriasis.

The diffuse form is generally met with in adults, and upon the extensor surfaces of the body or about the joints. It seldom attacks the palms of the hands or the soles of the feet, but when it does it is apt to be very obstinate. It occasionally attacks the nails, giving them a yellowish appearance, producing thickening, roughening and destroying their lustre.

The scaling in this disease, especially in the diffuse form, is sometimes very extensive. As the eruption disappears the scaling grows less, often disappearing, first from the centre, leaving marginal rings; finally the redness fades and the skin again resumes a normal appearance. Pruritus may be severe or only slight. Very often the general health of the patient is quite good, although a gouty diathesis is frequently present.

Pathology—The pathological lesion consists in an hypertrophy of the upper cutaneous layers of the skin.

Etiology—Psoriasis is met with at all ages, and in both sexes. It is found more frequently between the ages of ten and thirty years, and in the gouty and rheumatic, or in those patients having a marked uric acid diathesis.

The extensive use of meats, meat extracts, rich broths, etc., tends to develop this disease.

Prognosis—All uncomplicated cases are curable under good homœopathic treatment.

REMEDIES—Arum, Ars., Iod. ars., Calc., Dulc., Graph., Iod., Lyc., Mer. sol., Nitr. ac., Petr, Phos., Psor., Sep., Sulph., Teucr., Tub., Medorrh.

PART V

CLASSIFICATION—NEW GROWTHS

This classification of diseases of the skin embraces a class of diseases that are as varied in their nature as in their number. They include all those false structures and new formatious from the simple bridge builder, the cicatricial white fibrous tissue, to that of lupus and even true cancer. When we speak of "New Growths" we do not mean new, healthy, normal tissue growths, but a false growth. We mean that some power is added to the life force, some perversion of action has taken place, not within the cell or the local tissue alone, but within the life force itself, within the vitalizing principle, giving it the power to make false things from false material foreign to the organism; in other words, that power that produces new growths is an over-action, and, sooner or later, an over-action means death of the part or of the whole organism. At no better place can we learn that great truth, made known to the world by Hahnemann, that "Disease is disturbance of the Life Force," and that disturbance is due wholly to a morbific agent, a subversive force known as a miasm, either as psora, or some other miasm in combination with psora. Psora, however taken by itself, seldom gives us a true malignancy; always do we fiind sycosis, or syphilis, or both together accompanying it in new growths. Therefore, in our study of new growths let us keep in mind that a new growth, which is a false growth, must have as a primary predisposing cause, psora in combination with some other miasms as a basis. If more than two miasms are present, the greater is the possibility, not only of a malignancy, but a rapid and destructive one. Psora and syphilis together will in time give us the true tubercular diathesis. Now infect that organism with the sycotic poison, and watch the new vigor a malignancy receives by its presence. The life force seems to have received a new power to destroy life so frequently seen in malignant phthisis, lupus vulgaris and true cancer.

I know of no class of diseases by which the student of medicine can study the action of the miasms to better advantage than in this class of diseases, where the vital forces are so profoundly disturbed, and the life processes so changed in their action, or where the phenomena pre sented are so unique, positive, and persistent.

New growths may involve any or all the structures of the skin, or they may, in the later stages of the disease, dip down into the connective tissue, and even the deeper organs lying beneath.

CICATRIX (Scar)

A cicatrix is a new connective tissue formation covered with epithelium, without which it cannot be called a true scar. A cicatrix takes the place of normal skin that has been in some way destroyed. It only takes place where there is a destruction of the cutis, especially the papillary layer. If the epithelial layer only is destroyed it will not scar. Shallow scars in time disappear, but deep ones remain permanent. They show no pores, hairs, glands, or organs of the skin present, but they have papillæ and a thin epithelial layer on their surface. They are usually smooth, but they may be ridged and uneven, movable, or fixed and anchored to the underlying tissue. New scars are reddish or pinkish in color, but old ones are usually smooth, shiny, and sometimes glistening. They are said to be flat when on the level of the skin, atrophic when depressed, and hypertrophic when elevated above the surface. Microscopically, we find them composed of connective tissue bundles interlacing each other, as if woven together. While young they are richly supplied with bloodvessels, but as they become aged, only scantily supplied. The so-called scars of pregnancy are not a true cicatrix, but are due to a distension of these fibrous connective tissue bundles.

Scars are divided into pathological and traumatic, or those from injury and those from disease.

Pathology—They are often of great diagnostic value; of course, the younger they are the easier the cause or origin of the lesion is to determine. They are linear in incised wounds that heal by first intention, irregular after burns and ulceration. After prolonged or suppurative processes the surrounding tissue is more or less pigmented, indurated, or in some way shows an inflammatory process of long duration. Tubercular ulceration leaves an irregular and extensive scar, while the scars of lupus are superficial. Syphilitic scars usually show the peculiar brownish or copper-colored pigmentation for a long time, and sometimes it is permanently present, presenting bean-shaped, horse-shoe, round or oval, depressed lesions with sharp, well-defined edges. They occasionally deform or distort the affected part, as seen in burns. or produce pain occasionally by pressure.

KELOID

DEFINITION—Keloid is a circumscribed connective tissue new growth, of which there are two forms: the false and the true.

The former develops from an old scar, and the latter without any previous injury to the skin.

Symptomatology—The disease begins in small bean-sized nodules or tumors imbedded deeply, yet slightly elevated above the surface of the skin. The nodules are smooth, with radiating roots, or projections from their margin. The disease progresses slowly, with very little change in the color of the skin. If any change in the color, it becomes pale and bleached. The affection begins spontaneously, with no apparent cause, or is due to traumatism or from an old scar. We recall two marked keloids occurring on the back of a young lady that were induced by the use of a strong electric current. At first it produced a slight cautery, which developed within a year to keloid. They are also known to follow nervous disorder.

Etiology—The etiology is unknown. It is found to be more prevalent in the African race; also, in those tubercular patients who have deep-seated nervous troubles. They have been known to develop from slight surgical operations from traumatism, and from an old cicatrix.

Pathology—They are a dense connective tissue growth.

Diagnosis—They have nothing in common except it be the disease known as morphea.

Prognosis—It is a slow and difficult disease to cure, and occasionally may have to be referred to surgery.

Treatment—Cures are reported to have been made with Caust., Nit. ac., Sil., Graph., Sabina, Fluor. ac., Psor., Tub.

Probably more cures are made, however, with Fluoric acid than any other remedy. Cal. carb., Sil., Fluor. ac., Psor., Tub., Sulph., Sil. are frequently indicated.

MALIGNANT "NEW GROWTHS"

Epithelioma—DEFINITION—A malignant epithelial new growth which undergoes ulceration, and which returns after removal by surgical or local methods.

Symptomatology—Three forms or varieties present themselves for study: The superficial, deep seated and the papillary.

SUPERFICIAL—The superficial or discoid form is a semi-malignant form of carcinoma involving the skin and mucous membrane. The disease seldom presents itself before the age of forty or fifty, the primary lesion making its appearance in the form of a very small, pale red or waxy, glistening, flat-topped, semi-transparent papule. It is single at times, but generally grouped with from three to six papules in a group, looking very much like smooth, flat warts on the surface of the skin. They may remain in this form for years. The first change, however, is a slight fissuring across their surfaces, with a slight, scarcely perceptible hæmorrhage at times. Later on it exudes a thin, scanty, light colored tenacious secretion which dries into a thin, brownish crust. What is peculiar about this apparently very simple abrasion of the skin is that it shows no disposition to heal. A microscopic examination reveals epithelial cells of various forms and sizes. As the disease advances, which is generally slow, the superficial lesion increases, and finally breaks down into a superficial ulcer. The edges of the ulcer become well defined, and the surrounding tissue soon becomes infiltrated, and the glands sympathetically affected. The destruction continues upon the surface of the skin. Sometimes it is so superficial as to involve only the papillary layer of the derma, healing in the center while it spreads at the periphery; again it involves the deeper structures until the greater part of the face or scalp may be implicated, and death results from exhaustion or the production of *metastatic* growths in the different organs.

DEEP SEATED—The deep seated or infiltrating form

may arise from the simple lesion, but it generally begins as a nodule in the connective tissue, or from an old wart that is undergoing degenerative changes. This nodule is usually of the size of a common bean and of a purplish-red color, with a congested areola, elevated some above the surface of the skin, slightly sensitive to touch, but not painful in the beginning. Sooner or later it breaks down into an irregular-shaped ulcer with steep and everted walls. Its floor is covered with a yellowish, offensive secretion, bleeding easily when touched, and showing rapid infiltration into the surrounding tissues. Pain is usually present, of a sharp lancinating character. The neighboring glands become involved and the patient's symptoms grow from bad to worse, until the whole system succumbs to the influence of malignancy, dying usually from exhaustion. The secretion from this form of the disease is abundant, thin, of a dirty yellowish-green watery consistency, of a dreadfully offensive odor. Sometimes it dries into a brownish crust.

Complication: Stasis to internal organs, acute inflammatory diseases, hæmorrhages, and exhaustion from septic processes.

Diagnosis—The diagnosis is not difficult when we consider the age of the patient, the odor and general nature of the discharges, the persistence and the destructive processes of the disease.

Papillary Epithelioma—This form is usually met with on the mucous membrane, but more frequently on the peripheral border, between the mucous membrane and the skin, although it may appear on the scrotum, the extremities and other parts. Papilla usually develop upon the surface of the ulcer, increasing until it has a condylomatous appearance. It is very vascular, bleeds easily and profusely at times, early and rapidly involves the deeper structures and glands. The symptoms that follow are similar to those of the deep-seated form, the average duration of life seldom exceeding three or four years.

LUPUS ERYTHEMATOSUS

Erythematosus Lupus

This form of lupus is even now considered by some authors to be not of tubercular origin, but the bacillus has been found in sufficient numbers to establish the fact that it is. The disease begins with an inflammation or patch of redness round the opening of a sebaceous gland. which gradually spreads. Its surface becomes scaly, the margin well defined and slightly raised. These patches or spots run together in time and new ones form in the progress of the disease. They are dark or bright red in color, slightly elevated, somewhat shiny, covered with scales or crusts, although the latter are usually absent. The sebaceous glands are usually plugged up, and often the orifices of the glands are obliterated. The amount of scaling varies greatly in the different cases. These little patches may remain stationary for years, but gradually their borders fade, and they undergo atrophic changes, leaving scars. The seat of the disease is usually upon the nose, face, scalp, although it may occur on other parts of the body. There are no constitutional symptoms, and the local symptoms are often confined to slight itching and burning. The general health of the patient usually remains good.

Diagnosis—The diagnostic points are: The location, the round, red, slightly elevated disks. The central scarring and its chronic tendency; the absence of constitutional symptoms. It seldom occurs before the age of puberty.

Pathology—It is a chronic tubercular inflammation of the cutis, involving the sebaceous glands, which leads to their degeneration and atrophy.

Treatment—Agar., Alum., Ars., Calc., Carbol. ac., Caust., Cist. can., Graph., Guararco, Hep., Sulph., Psor., Hydrocotyle, Kali c., Kali b., Nit. ac., Phyto., Rhus tox., Sep., Staph., Sil., Medorrh., Tub., Lupus, Lach., Lac can.

LUPUS VULGARIS

Lupus vulgaris is another new cell growth of the skin, and is now included under the tubercular skin affections. It first makes its appearance upon the skin in the form of small pin-head-sized, soft, reddish papules or tubercles, either isolated or grouped together, yet not touching each other. They usually coalesce, developing into patches. These patches increase in size by the further development of new tubercles upon their periphery. These tubercles are indolent, soft, elastic, and occasionally sensitive to pressure; their progress of change is slow, but sooner or later they break down and ulcerate. The ulcers are generally round, shallow excavations, with reddish granulations covering their base. They secrete a thin and often offensive secretion, which dries into a thin, dry crust. The edges are soft and bleed easily. A slow destructive, ulcerative process continues beneath these crusts. They are seldom sensitive or painful. The tubercular bacilli are rarely found, but the micro-organisms of suppuration are present in great numbers. Sometimes the ulcer takes on a vegetative character or papillary fungoid growth.

Lupus Papillaris—(Verrucous)—This form generally develops upon the nose, and produces by its ulcerative and destructive process great deformity, even the complete destruction of the organ. Lupus vulgaris often makes its appearance soon after puberty, occurring more frequently in females. It involves the skin, mucous membrane, and cartilage, never affecting the osseous structure. When the disease is well established, all stages of the disease may be manifest at the same time, presenting papules or new tubercles just making their appearance, or older ones undergoing softening, or ulcerative processes, ulcers, crusts, scars, etc.

The lupus ulcer may develop symmetrically, or it may take on a serpiginous form, which spreads in some particular direction, sometimes causing marked deformity, and noted for its persistent chronic course and its resistance to treatment. The disease occurs more frequently upon the nose, lips, face, cheeks, and ears, but may occur upon other parts of the body.

Diagnosis—It is to be distinguished from syphilis, lupus erythematosis, epithelioma, acne, rosacea, and eczema squamosum. From syphilis it is distinguished by its early history and the general progress of the two affections, the lupus ulceration being slow, and the syphilitic ulcer undergoing more rapid changes. Besides in lupus there is a tendency for the ulcer to heal; also, in lupus there are thin brownish crusts, while in syphilis the crusts are thick, dark green, with profuse, purulent discharge, the scars being smooth, white, and circumscribed. Epithelioma begins in middle life, is more painful and more rapid in its development. It is accompanied with hæmorrhages, involves neighboring lymphatics and the deeper structures, is always single, and cicatrix does not form. Lupus erythematosus also begins in adult life, and consists of red papules or disks; never ulcerates; is covered with scales, and involves the sebaceous follicles. In squamous eczema there is no ulceration and no discharge.

Diagnosis—The early history of its beginning, its location upon the face, the color and shape of the ulcer, the tendency to heal, its absence of subjective symptoms. A microscopic examination should always be made, to assist in confirming the diagnosis.

Treatment—Lupus in General. Remedies: Agar., Alum., Ant. crud., Ars., Bar. c., Cal. c., Carbol. ac., Caust., Cist. can, Graph., Kali c., Kali bich., Kali iod., Nit. ac., Rhus tox., Sep., Sil., Staph., Sulph., Aurum mur., Uranium, Thuja, Calotropis, Hydrocot., Lyc., Tub., Psor., Phos., Luperinum guarana, Hyd., Oleum jac. an., Nat. mur., Lach., Lac can., Carb. veg., Carb. an., Asaf., Kali sulph., Mez., Ars. iod., Phyt., Bufo, Kreo., Con., Iod., Mer., Therid., Zinc., Zinc. phos., Cal. fl., Dul., Lill., Medorrh., Pet., Sanic, Secal., Sars., Syph., X-ray.

INDICATIONS—*Arsenicum alb.*—Foul, destructive ulcer: discharge thin, watery, excoriating the parts passed over. Face pale, sallow, sometimes waxy; anxious expression of countenance, ulcers with hard edges, with much burning; if there is pain it is worse at night, after 1 P. M. In later stages thirst with rapid emaciation; crusts thin brown.

Apis—Small ulcers, with grayish sluff. Skin colorless, waxy, no thirst (Ars., thirst), relieved by cool bathing, edema, part much puffed and swollen; pain burning and stinging.

Aurum—Indicated in low-spirited, despondent people; discharge greenish, ichorous, putrid, syphilitic or Mercury patients; affects the nose and deeper structures of the face (Amm.); bone pains, worse at night (Mer., Syph., Nit., Kali iod.). Lesion brownish or yellow, ulcer deep, destructive, mental symptoms of a suicidal nature; dark haired, lively, restless people who when ill are despondent and suicidal.

Condurango—Malignant, open, foul smelling, destructive ulcers, with stinging, burning pains (Ars., Apis); scrofulous, syphilitic or tubercular individuals.

Graphites—Tubercular people, inclined to obesity, Lupus of face or nose; fissures and cracks that bleed easily. Sticky, honey-like secretion (Pet., Tub.); nails hard, horny, brittle; erysipelas following lupus.

Tuberculinum—Indicated in the early stages of both lupus and epithelioma; many cures made in the first stage and beginning of the second stage of epithelioma; very few symptoms; tubercles dry, hard, having small, fine fissures in the lesion that bleed easily (profusely, Nit. ac.).

Nitric acid—Bil. mot. temp. Clean cut ulcer, bleeds easily on being touched; vegetations; bleed at slightest touch; sticking, splintery-like pains in the ulcer; urine offensive; suitable to dark complected people with black hair and eyes; gnawing pains in ulcers; base of ulcer looks raw; discharges thin, offensive, acrid, dirty yellowish-green color; < evening and after midnight.

Guarana—Lupus of an ochre-red color; yellow spots on the face and temples.

Psorinum—Lupus following suppressed diseases; ulcers, eczema, psoriasis, scabies, skin dry, scaly; discharges very offensive, carrion-like; patients always chilly; takes cold easily; perspiration and all secretions offensive; > by warmth in general, by perspiration and in the summer.

LEPROSY (Scaly)

Leprosy is a chronic disease of the skin, now quite fully understood to be of tubercular origin, which may be inherited or acquired.

Symptomatology—Leprosy is one of the most ancient of diseases. It was ancient long before Moses wrote of the white spot upon the skin, 1490 years before the advent of Christ. If on examination of the diseased one there was found to be a white crusting, he was unclean, but if the scab was dark he was considered clean. It was called "The Plague of Leprosy," and to be infected with the disease in the slightest way was to be called "unclean, unclean." To be a possessor of that well known scaly spot or patch was to be doomed to death sooner or later, and to be despised by all men, and set apart forever.

The disease is usually divided into two forms, the tubercular and the anesthetic. They may differ only at times in the different stages of the disease, or in the tissues involved. Its distribution is very wide, including India, China, Japan and the majority of the islands of the Pacific and Indian Oceans. It is also found in the West Indies, South America, Mexico and sporadic cases in Scotland and in almost every country on the globe. It appears in Oriental countries either endemic or epidemic, usually, however, endemic.

The disease cannot be said to be directly or immediately contagious, as later investigation, as in the life of Father Damien among the Hawaiians, has shown, also by the testimony of many physicians who have followed up the history of special cases, we learn that it is necessary for the affected one to be in contact with the disease for some time, often for years.

The systemic invasion is a matter of years rather than months, constituting the period of incubation. However, when it is established, it often progresses rapidly.

The initial lesion, or the part to be first attacked is, in the majority of cases, according to Morrow, in the nasal passages, beginning in some form of rhinitis; an increased secretion or epistaxis is usually the first manifestation. A dry catarrh, circumscribed at first, followed by erythematous spots of a reddish brown or dark yellowish color, appearing in different parts of the body.

TUBERCULAR FORM

SYMPTOMS—The first symptom noticeable is a slight difficulty in breathing through the nose. The throat, larynx and nose symptoms are said to be present in about sixty per cent. of the cases. Later on localized nodosities appear in different parts of the body, more particularly on the face and hands; they are in size from that of a pea to a chestnut, and even larger. The cutis becomes hardened, thickened, or puckered, showing ridges or furrows. The hairs change in color often becoming white, and later on fall out. Pigmented spots appear on the thickened, hardened and knotty surfaces; in other nodules ulceration takes place. The ulcers are small, deep, with edges indurated and sharp cut, as in syphilis. As they proceed in their ravages they destroy every tissue even to the osseous structures, mucous membranes of the mouth, tongue, larynx, pharynx, nose, nasal cartilages and bones. The disease progresses slowly, however, 10 or 15 years is an average, interspersed with periods of febrile exacerbations or of comparative quiet. Great mutilation often takes place in the joints, toes, fingers, etc. Loss of the small joints of the fingers and toes is often unattended with pain. The general health gradually sinks under the disease until the patient dies from an involvement of some internal organ, either as an extension or intercurrent disease.

Ocular complications in both forms are numerous. In the anesthetic form, lag-ophthalmos, xerosis of the conjunctiva and iritis, cataract, and phthisis bulbi are frequent complications. In the tuberculous variety the cornea and conjunctiva are the chief seats of the lesion, although sometimes the iris, lens and whole eyeball become affected. Mental disorders, as melancholia, tubercular meningitis, nodular tuberculosis of the cerebellum and degeneration of the posterior column of the spinal cord are some of the severer complications.

Diagnosis—From tuberculosis it is differentiated by the absence of anesthetic areas and by the bacillus.

From syphilis the course of the disease and the history of syphilis, when gradually the patient succumbs to an invasion of the viscera or some intercurrent disease, pneumonia or some inflammatory process.

Anesthetic Leprosy—In this variety the spots are not so numerous, beginning usually in the palms of hands and soles of feet, resembling, however, the tubercular. Hyperæsthesia usually precedes the anesthesia over the hyperemic or diseased areas. The leprous spots do not, it is said, always correspond to the distribution of the nerves, but may spread in all directions. As the disease advances the anesthesia manifests itself, when it often becomes so marked that pricks of pins, even burns, are not felt by the patient. Pains are sometimes present of a shooting character; paralysis not uncommon.

Etiology—The disease is but slightly contagious. It requires often years to become affected, and that usually by a residence with the infected ones. It is no more due to a bacillus than any other disease, but to the disease syphilis ingrafted upon a peculiar psoric base, producing that strange tubercular process. The disease affects both sexes alike, being most frequently met with between twenty and forty years of age.

Treatment—Prophylaxis. Isolation is probably the only safe and sure prophylaxis. Sea bathing has been found beneficial. Chaulmugra oil in doses of one-half drachm daily has done considerable good in the leprosy hospital of Trinidad. Gurjun oil, from a tree growing in East India, has also been considerably used in the Philippines.

REMEDIES—Ars. alb., Ars. iod., Alum., Sep., Sulph., Psor., Tub., Amm. carb., Cal. c., Carbo veg., Caust., Con., Graph., Cup., Iod., Kali c., Lach., Lyc., Merc. sol., Phos., Sep., Sil., Still. sylv., Syph., Sulph., Zinc., Phos., Psor.

TUBERCULAR NEW GROWTHS

Rodent Ulcer. Ulcus Exedens

SYMPTOMS—The disease begins as a soft, brown tubercle upon the face, which may remain unchanged for years, but between the age of forty and fifty years the tubercle is liable to break down into an ulcer. Occasionally these tubercles or nodules increase to the size of a common chestnut before breaking down. One of the distinguishing features between this ulcer and an epithelial growth is the marked disproportion between the ulcer and the growth itself; the ulcerative process being more marked. There is very little pain, generally a scanty discharge, and it seldom involves the lymphatics; slowly and persistently, however, it destroys the part affected, producing great and unsightly deformities.

TUBERCULOSIS OF THE SKIN

In the study of tuberculosis of the skin a number of forms are to be presented that seem very diverse in their nature; in fact, they are quite foreign to each other, although classified in this family of diseases.

The strong resemblance of tubercular diseases of the skin to syphilis in its many variations is generally observed, but there are reasons for this when we come to study the tubercular and the syphilitic cell together. From a microscopic standpoint they are identical. Koch has observed this, and frequently calls our attention to the fact in his writings. Tuberculosis in all its varied and innumerable forms had its origin primarily in the tertiary tubercular syphilitic manifestation, which, being implanted upon the psoric base with its countless and varied changes, could not do therwise, each being endowed with a specific potential, than to produce just such changes and conditions as are seen in tuberculosis cutis. Lupus, tuberculosis, verricosa scrofula derma, leprosy, and, in fact, many other lesions and diseases of the skin, as well as of the organism in general, are now considered to be tubercular, that in the past were not so considered. A closer study of these conditions with the light thrown over them by modern methods of investigation reveal many things that show us that the cause of all disease, by no means, lies, as it appears, upon the surface, and that when we refer the causes of diseases to foods, climatic conditions, vocation and other external causes we come far short of the mark. Therefore, in our study of these diseases let us not confine ourselves to the histologic elements, the bacillus, or the histologic structure of these lesions alone; but let us consider them from the standpoint of a miasmatic basis, looking for the miasms of syphilis, psora and sycosis. This knowledge is of vital importance to the homœopathic physician in laying the foundation of our therapeutic superstructure. For we may say we have no perfect knowledge of any diseased condition until we have discovered its miasmatic basis, which alone reveals to us cause in its true light.

TUBERCULOSIS CUTIS

This form is of rare occurrence, known only to phthisical patients. The lesions are shallow ulcers found at the juncture of the mucous membrane and the skin around the orifices of the body. The floor of the ulcer shows miliary nodules, also about its periphery, and is bathed with a purulent secretion.

They are quite painful, due much, of course, to their location, and may be single or multiple. They continue a slow chronic course, causing much suffering to the individual. Secondary infection and involvement of the lungs, intestines, glands or, in fact, any organ may follow in the course of this disease. Sometimes, however, the ulcers are secondary, appearing in advanced stages of phthisis.

TUBERCULOSIS VERRUCOSA

Tuberculosis verrucosa is an affection of the hands, fingers, wrists, forearms of persons working in autopsy rooms, butchers, cooks, and those handling animal products. These patients are, as a rule, in good health.

The disease makes its appearance in the form of plaques of different sizes upon the backs of the hands. Sometimes they show marked inflammatory processes; again these are found wanting. The lesions begin as tubercles of a soft consistency, which take on a form of papillary hypertrophy; it runs a chronic course, often lasting for years, undergoing very little alteration, but later on in the disease the lymphatic system may become affected. and the tubercular affection extend to deeper structures or to internal organs.

SCROFULA DERMA

DEFINITION—A tubercular process of the subcutaneous tissue, involving the skin only secondarily.

SYMPTOMS—The lesions usually occur upon the face and neck, but may develop on other portions of the body, especially the chest and back. It is only a form of that general strumous condition so liable to develop in tubercular cases. The lesions appear in dull, reddish, soft, tubercular formations that soon suppurate, and are covered with dark crusts, from beneath which oozes yellowish green tubercular pus. In the ulcerative process unhealthy granulations often spring up which bleed freely when touched or irritated, and when the healing process takes place they leave ugly looking scars.

Other tubercular processes may be present, such as onychia, ulceration of mucous surfaces, lymphatic involvement with abscesses.

Diagnosis—The diagnosis is made from the general diathesis of the patient. It differs from a syphilitic process by the absence of pigmentation; the superficial character of the ulcer, its history and its slow chronic course.

Etiology—True it is not syphilis alone; but it is true that all tubercular processes arise from latent syphilis engrafted upon a psoric base. In lupus we must add to it sycosis, when a close study will reveal the presence of all three miasms.

TUMORS

FIBROMA

DEFINITION—Fibroma of the skin is a connective tissue NEW GROWTH. There are two forms, the hard and the soft, depending upon the character of the connective tissue. The former generally appears singly, and the latter multiple. They develop from the lower layers of the cutis and the connective tissue. The hard form occurs upon the trunk and extremities; sometimes on the face. They are smooth, oval or round, occurring at any age; grow slowly, are quite small in size, usually from that of a pinhead to that of a pea, but may grow larger. They seldom become malignant, generally ending in calcification. The soft form, sometimes called molluscum, are sessile, pedunculated, circumscribed, covered by normal skin. In size they are from a split pea and even smaller to that of a hen's egg, but they may grow to a great size. A few cases are reported where they weighed as high as from ten to forty pounds. The small tumors are only felt beneath the skin as little nodules. Traumatism of any kind hastens their growth, which is generally very slow They may appear in any portion of the body, but the eyelids, face and head are favored locations.

Etiology—Etiology is unknown.

Pathology—Microscopically, they have been found to be of a myxomatous character or partially of the fibrous element and partially of myxomatous element.

Prognosis—Favorable.

Treatment—Surgical in long standing cases, but many cases can be cured with our remedies.

LIPOMA (Fatty Tumor)

DEFINITION—An adipose growth of the skin and connective tissue.

SYMPTOMS—The fatty tumor presents itself in two forms: the diffuse and the circumscribed, the latter occuring more frequently. The former is flattened and lobulated, and the circumscribed round and pear-shaped, from the size of a hickory nut upwards to that of an orange, or larger. The skin over these growths is movable, normal in color, although sometimes pigmented. They develop slowly or remain stationary for years. They present no subjective symptoms, except occasional pain from pressure. They are of a soft, doughy feeling to the touch.

Pathology—They are composed of adipose and connective tissue elements. They grow to a certain size, then usually remain stationary. Some cases show calcareous deposits. It is said that the circumscribed forms occur more frequently in women, while the diffuse lypoma occurs oftener in males. They are both a growth of adult life.

Diagnosis—The absence of pain or subjective symptoms; the lobular, soft, doughy-like, rounded tumor makes the diagnosis easy.

Treatment—Surgical and medicinal. We recall two cases of lypoma of the back, both in women over forty years of age, each removed by an operation, when soon after similar growths developed in close proximity to the former, that were cured by Silica c. m., the treatment extending over a period of fourteen months. In these patients it was clearly shown that their life force was in such an abnormal condition that it must create tumors, and not until that false physiological process was destroyed by the indicated homœopathic remedy could it cease that abnormal action.

MYOMA

Myoma is a rare form of new growth. The tumors are pea or cherry sized, round or oval, of a purplish or pale red color, occurring single or multiple; located in the scrotum in men, or in the labia majora or nipples in women. They occur at any age. They are usually without symptoms but may be painful.

Pathology—They are composed of muscle fibre and connective tissue elements.

Diagnosis—The diagnosis is often quite difficult, and may have to be settled by a microscope.

Prognosis—Prognosis good.

NEUROMA (Nerve Tumor)

The neuroma is composed of nerve fibre, is very small in size, never, as a rule, growing larger than a hazel nut, occurring single or multiple, partially movable with the skin, of a pinkish color, and situated in the corium, extending into the subcutaneous tissue. It occurs at any time of life, but generally at middle or old age. In their early history they are not painful, but later on are very painful; the pain taking on that of a paroxysmal nature, being greatly aggravated by change of weather.

Diagnosis—Diagnosis is often difficult, as it resembles other growths. The character of the pain is, however, of great assistance in the diagnosis.

Etiology—To the pathologist the cause of the neuroma, as in all other cases of tumor, is an invisible thing that cannot be followed up to any source, therefore unknown.

Treatment—A careful study of our therapeutic armamentarium is all that is necessary in the cure of these simple yet very annoying growths.

ANGIOMA

Synonym—Vascular nevis.

Definition—Angioma is a new growth composed of bloodvessels and lymphatics.

Symptoms—They are usually congenital or appear soon

after birth. They are round, irregular, flat, or elevated above the skin; of a bright red or bluish color, and in size from that of a mustard seed and upwards to that of the hand, sometimes involving large surfaces or areas, varying in shade and color, smooth, or transversed with tortuous and dilated vessels, occasionally very vascular, and showing the pulsation of the bloodvessels. They occur more frequently on the head, face, lips, or other parts of the body. They may appear alone or in multiple; sometimes their surfaces are covered with warty-like growths, or deeply pigmented. By pressure they are deprived of their color which, when relieved, it immediately resumes. They may remain stationary for years or for a life time; sometimes, however, they increase in size; seldom do they take on a malignant nature. Where large surfaces are involved the outlines are quite irregular in form, with a blackberry stain or port wine color. They are seldom accompanied with any subjective symptoms, or rarely ever in any way inconvenience the patient, except it be from their appearance as a deformity, especially if about the head or face.

Pathology—They are situated in the upper part of the corium and connective tissue, and are composed of dilated and hypertrophied bloodvessels and the connective tissue element.

Diagnosis—The different shaped, flat, or elevated macules or patches with their network of tortuous vessels, their color, persistence, and freedom from subjective symptoms.

Etiology—The pathologist gives us no light upon the subject whatever. They are without doubt of sycotic origin.

Treatment—The treatment of tumors will be considered under lupus and malignant growths.

PART VI

CLASSIFICATION—HÆMORRHAGES

Cutaneous hæmorrhages into the cutis may take place in many ways. There are two forms to be especially considered: The idiopathic and the symptomatic; those occurring from the effects of injuries are known as idiopathic, and those occurring from the effects of internal diseases symptomatic. The hæmorrhage may occur by external injury to a bloodvessel itself, or the blood may escape through the capillary walls into the skin. Four special lesions are recognised: Vibices, petechia, ecchymosis, ecchymomata. The first mentioned occurs in narrow lines or streaks; the second in small spots differing in form and size from that of a pin-head to that of a dime, frequently seen in typhoid fever and other eruptive diseases of an inflammatory nature; the third form is where the hæmorrhage is more extensive and copious, appearing in large patches; the fourth is where it occurs in tumors or elevated patches. The idiopathic hæmorrhage is the result of injuries induced by wounds, bruises, contusions or from insect bites and stings; may also be the result of certain drugs.

The symptomatic arises from systemic disturbances alone, such as small-pox, typhoid fever, also other forms of fever; from urticaria, pemphigus, rheumatism, and gouty states of the system, even certain forms of hysteria has been known to be followed with some form of purpura. Hæmorrhagic diseases are not so much a disease of the skin as they are due to diseases of the bloodvessels, directly as in external injuries, or indirectly to systemic disturbances. Hæmorrhages of the skin have occurred occasionally through the medium of perspiration (bloody sweat), also in vicarious menstruation. The pathological changes due to hæmorrhages into the skin are all classified under what is known as *purpura*, and more especially those forms due to symptomatic causes, which may appear in one or more of the lesions mentioned.

PURPURA (Purple Spots)

Three forms of purpura present themselves for consideration: Purpura simplex, purpura rheumatica, and purpura hæmorrhagica.

Purpura Simplex—Purpura simplex may be defined as a slightly elevated purple spot or patch upon the skin, differing in form and size, and which does not disappear upon pressure.

SYMPTOMS—It may occur as petechia, vibices, or ecchymosis, seldom having any constitutional symptoms, and usually without any previous warning, occasionally slight malaise or chilliness. The disease generally appears suddenly, occurring in any part of the body, and in size from a mere speck to that of a split pea, and more frequently upon the extremities, usually multiple. There are no objective symptoms except a slight soreness. Wheals or vesicles may arise as a complication. The spots usually disappear within ten or twelve days.

Purpura Rheumatica—DEFINITION.—A purpuric eruption accompanied with similar phenomena to that of acute rheumatism.

SYMPTOMS—The premonitory symptoms are lassitude, headache, loss of appetite and general bad feeling; usually swelling of one or more of the joints, with more or less severe pain of a rheumatic character, which may be either localized or general. This is accompanied with fever, restlessness and the general suffering as found in acute rheumatism. Frequently do we witness this condition of things, lasting from three to five days, feeling quite sure of our diagnosis to be acute rheumatism, only to find between the third and fifth day a purpuric eruption, quite general over the body, more marked upon the extremities and abdomen, with a gradual subsidence of the fever, pain and other symptoms, and within a week the patient is convalescent. The spots are generally about the size of the finger nails, and do not disappear on pressure. At first of a reddish or purplish hue, which soon changes to a yellowish or greenish tinge, due to the natural processes of the effused blood. They are gradually absorbed and disappear, the fever and pain subsiding with the appearance of the eruption. Relapses are not uncommon, however, as is sometimes seen in acute rheumatism, and are occasionally accompanied with gastro-intestinal diseases. The disease occurs in both sexes, but more frequently in women.

Pathology—Rupture of a capillary vessel with fibrous clots, emboli and micro-organisms found in the transudate.

Etiology—The disease occurs more frequently in the early spring, in low bottoms where there is much dampness and poor drainage. The disease occurs, I think, only in rheumatic or gouty patients, or those having a sycotic taint.

Treatment—The treatment should in general follow that similarly employed in acute rheumatism.

Remedies—Acon., Arn., Ars., Bell., Bry., Bapt., Rhus tox., Ruta, Rhus rad., Chloral., Ham., Lach., Mer. c., Phos., Ver. vir., Lyc., Tart. em., Crotal., Led., Kalm., Dolich., Benzo. ac., Fer. phos., Puls., Amm. c., Colins,

Phyto., Bryonia, Pulsatilla and Arsenicum are frequently indicated.

Purpura Hæmorrhagica—A severe form of purpura, accompanied with marked constitutional symptoms a purpuric eruption upon the skin and frequently hæmorrhages from internal organs.

SYMPTOMS—Usually preceded by severe constitutional symptoms, gastric disturbances, fever and much prostration. Suddenly the hæmorrhagic spots appear upon the skin, first upon the extremities, then on other parts of the body, often to be followed by hæmorrhages from internal organs, mouth, nose, bowels and bladder, and effusions into the conjunctiva, choroid, as well as into the skin. It is always considered a very dangerous disease, death frequently occurring from heart failure, anæmia, hæmorrhages and exhaustion. Several times I have noticed in leukemia small bloodvessel rupture, and ecchymotic spots appear upon the skin within a few moments. The first sensation noticed by the patient being a slight stinging pain; also, blood tumors, the size of an egg, appeared upon the abdominal wall, or upon tne extremities, while at the same time the body was dotted over with purpuric spots. Purpura fulminans, although a rare disease, is the most to be dreaded of the hæmorrhagic forms, which often destroys life in twenty-four or forty-eight hours, beginning with a severe chill, followed by a high temperature from 106, or higher, accompanied with severe rheumatic pains, delirium, coma, collapse and death within a day or two.

REMEDIES—Ham., Ars., Rhus tox., Amm. mur., Lach., Carbo veg., Mur. ac., Nit. ac., Phos., Phos. ac., Tub., Bry., Secal., Croc., Ip., Sabina, Ustila., China off., Melilot., Fer. met., Alet., Hyos., Pyro.

Indication for purpura is general. Aconite in the early

stage of the rheumatic form of purpura where there is high fever with general restlessness, mental anxiety with fear, skin dry, hot, burning thirst.

Belladonna—(Bil-vital-temp.) Purpura rheumatica, and occasionally in the hæmorrhagic form; violent fever, drowsy, sleepy during fever; full, rapid pulse with dry, hot skin, which burns to the touch; pupils large, face red, eyes stary, glassy-like; great thirst for sips of water; mucous membrane of the mouth dry; hæmorrhages from the nose where the blood feels hot; eruptive fevers with petechia, violent delirium during the fever; attacks of pain very acute, especially in the joints; paroxysmal, coming and going suddenly.

Arsenicum—(Sang-ment-vit-temp.) Hæmorrhagic or rheumatic forms; great prostration with general loss of strength; patients anæmic, bloodless; hæmorrhages from internal organs, with great mental restlessness, anxiety and fear of dealth; unquenchable thirst for small sips of cold water, which frequently produce vomiting; anxious expression of the face, pale, sallow, waxy after hæmorrhages; patient is better by warmth and by lying down. Any purpuric lesion may be found under this remedy. The tongue is usually dry, white, or brown, with no moisture in the mouth (Bell.), constant desire to moisten the lips. Hæmorrhages from the bowels are dark and offensive; respiration quick, pulse feeble; patient constantly moaning and complaining; symptoms worse usually at one P. M.; black ecchymosis under the skin; petechia with miliary eruption; morbus maculosus; tendency to anasarca.

Arnica—(Bil-mot-temp.) Traumatic purpura due to falls, bruises, contusions, and injuries in general; purpura bluish, black, or bluish-green; very sensitive and tender to touch; sore, bruised feeling after internal hæmorrhages in injuries or from febrile states, or tired feeling as if beaten all over; purpuric spots tender and sore to touch; cannot bear to be moved on account of soreness.

Baptisia—(Bil-mot-lymph-temp.) Purpura hæmorrhagica of typhus, or typhoid fever, or small-pox; internal hæmorrhages during their course; tongue dry, cracks in fevers (Pyro.); can swallow liquids only; mental symptoms, indifference, stupor, falls to sleep while being spoken to, unable to fix the mind on anything; face dusky, dark, as if deeply intoxicated; sensation as if parts of the body were separated; stools dark brown, bloody; hæmorrhages dark, thin, watery and offensive.

Lachesis—(Bil-mot-lymp.) All forms of purpura; eruptions purplish, or black, usually very sensitive to touch (Arnica, Bell.); purpura with dark blebs or burning vesicles; body covered with red or bluish eruption; purpura with dark purple colored bullæ, sometimes gangrenous (Carbo veg., Secal.); hæmorrhages from internal organs black as ink; hæmorrhages with hot flushes, followed by perspiration (Sulph., Ferr.); blood black, thin, watery; symptoms all worse after sleep; small wounds bleed easily (Phos.); purpura from septic fevers or wounds.

China off—Passive forms of hæmorrhages (Ham., Croc., Fer. phos.). Stout, swarthy persons whose systems become broken down from hæmorrhages or loss of vital fluids; apathetic, indifferent people (Phos. ac.). Extreme prostration and great debility after hæmorrhages; weakness of the limbs; roaring or ringing in the ears; skin cold, clammy (Carbo veg., Ars.). Tendency to hæmorrhages; blood usually thin and dark, It is complementary to Fer. m.

Crocus sat—Hæmorrhages black, clotty, stringy.

Hæmorrhages with cold sweat and desire to be fanned (Carbo veg.). Purpuric spots with pricking and crawling of the skin; blood hangs in strings from bleeding surfaces.

Ferrum met—(Sang-temp.) Pale, anæmic people who frequently have flushing of the face; face and lips pale, even white, hæmorrhagic diathesis; blood bright red, coagulates easily (Dark, Crocus, Sabina, Lach., Ham.). (Blood red, Fer. phos.). Ferrum is very similar to Pulsatilla in its action; general relaxation and weakness of the whole muscular system; pale, bloated appearance of the skin, or sallow and dirty looking; purpura of violet color; vertigo and fainting after hæmorrhages, if they attempt to sit or stand.

Hamamelis—(Bil-mot-temp.) Passive hæmorrhages, and painless, from the skin or from any of the orifices of the body. No subjective symptoms except slight soreness; hæmorrhage dark, profuse, passive, non-coagulative. It is a, good remedy to follow Arnica or Bellis per. after injuries. It is complementary to Fer. m.

Bryonia — (Bil-motor-temp.) Purpura rheumatica; sharp, shooting, stinging pains in joints; worse by the slightest motion, desire to lie perfectly quiet; great thirst for large drinks of cold water; patient is cross and irritable, hard to please; purpuric spots size of the finger nail, worse on the extremities and abdomen; pains disappear as soon as the eruption appears. Purpura a reddish blue.

Carbo, veg.—(Bil-mot-temp.) Purpura or purpuric hæmorrhages in exhausting diseases; one of our best remedies for the bad effects of the loss of blood (China, Ars., Phos.) Hæmorrhages from any mucous surface; blood oozes continually; coldness of the extremities, knees, nose and ears after hæmorrhages, or cold sweat with general

12

collapse; desire for cold air or to be fanned; copious cold sweat; voice hoarse, almost lost; hæmorrhages dark colored, thin; purpuric spots dark blue or black; skin in general blue and cyanotic.

Muriatic acid—(Bill-mot-temp.) Persons with black hair, dark eyes and dark complexion; irritable, peevish patients; diseases of an asthenic type; unconsciousness or moaning in low forms of fever, with loss of muscular power; all diseases take on a malignant type, and all discharges are foul and offensive; tongue dry, shrunken, leather-like in low fevers, with petechia upon the skin, or purpura purplish-red, black in small-pox, with offensive pustules.

Secale cor—Purpura hæmorrhagica; purpuric spots ulcerate and become gangrenous, or malignant pustules form on the skin; the hæmorrhages are black, thin or lumpy; skin dry, cold; pulse small, quick; discharges thin, black, foul smelling; chronic passive hæmorrhages in scrawny, feeble, cachectic women; ecchymosis into the skin; blood blisters forming and becoming gangrenous; all diseases worse from heat, and better by cold and uncovering.

Phosphorus—(Bil-mental-temp.) Tall, thin, slender people who walk stooped (Sulph.). Hæmorrhages profuse, pouring out freely from nose, mouth, bowels. Tubercular patients who are subject to hæmorrhages; bleeding of the gums (Mer., Nit. ac.); blood very fluid, difficult to coagulate; purpura hæmorrhagica, small spots of extravasated blood all over the body; small wounds bleed profusely; hawks or spits up blood constantly; blood bright red; purpura with formication and itching of the affected part.

ELEPHANTIASIS

DEFINITION—A chronic epidemic or sporadic circumscribed hypertrophic disease of the skin, involving the subcutaneous connective tissue, with inflammation, embolus of the blood and lymphatic channels, resulting in great swelling, edema and marked induration with pigmentation, and sometimes accompanied with fissures and warty growths.

SYMPTOMS—The legs are most frequently involved, but the genitals of both sexes usually follow closely, while any other part of the body may become affected. It is said to attack the right leg more frequently than the left, but both may be affected.

In the male the scrotum is next in frequency, and in the female the labia and clitoris. In India it sometimes occurs as an epidemic disorder, but is commonly a sporadic disease. The prodromal stage differs in the different climates. In hot climates there is usually a fever known as the elephantoid fever, preceded by severe pains in the lumbar region, often with retching and vomiting; coldness and shivering along the spine, followed with fever and profuse perspiration. In colder climates, however, it is not marked by such symptoms. Sometimes there is no pain or suffering whatever; but usually there are recurrent attacks of dermatitis of an erysipelatous character, the bacteria of erysipelas being found in some cases. Inflammation with chylous discharges are often met with. The deeper tissues become affected later on and these recurrent attacks may be weeks or months apart, or quite close together; each leaves the affected part, however, increased in size, until it becomes a colossal enlargement. The skin of the surface becomes waxy, pigmented, brownish, pinkish-red, or a deep sepia color, and on its surface sebaceous secretions, fissures, hard or soft tubercles, deep sulci; occasionally the tubercles bleed or present an eczematous appearance;

even ulceration may be present. All the tissues, even the osseous structures, later on share in the enlargement, until the size and weight of the part is out of all proportion to the body; pains of a sticking, stabbing, or boring nature are now quite constant, and headache, gastric disturbances, and sometimes delirium are present; and the suffering of these patients at times is past conception. Some of the severest forms are met with in the Oriental or in the African races.

Diagnosis—Early in the disease it is often difficult, but the recurrent erysipelatous attacks of inflammation confined to the same part, together with the gradual chronic enlargement, make the diagnosis easy.

Pathology—Changes in the subcutaneous tissue are marked. Upon cutting open the tissues, a yellowish grayish mass is exposed, showing in places lardaceous or fatty deposits exuding lymph. All the tissues share in the enlargement and infiltration, which is, of course, due to obstruction. Sporadic types in which the obstruction is induced by tumor-pressure, or other forms of pressure on the lymph or bloodvessels, develop about the same phenomena, yet they are quite easily distinguished.

Etiology—It occurs in all countries, climates and conditions of men, yet no certain cause has as yet been settled upon. Like all other diseases, its cause is not finite; no cause can be finite outside of the mechanical or chemical; therefore, cause is an infinite thing, and lies within the life force itself, latent and hereditary often; subject to development into some form of disease, depending on the nature of that internal dynamis and its external influences, be they dietetic, hygienic, atmospheric, electrothermal or planetary.

Prognosis—Always guarded, yet climate, hygiene, diet,

surgical and therapeutic means do much for these sufferers; curing some and greatly modifying others.

Treatment—No special indications can well be given in this disease. However, the following remedies are to be studied: Anac., Alum., Ars., Calotrophis., Carica., Jalapa, Graph., Hydrocotyle, Amm. mur., Apis, Lach., Pet,, Phos., Psor., Nat. carb., Nat. mur., Sepia, Sulph., Tub.

PART VII

CLASSIFICATION—ATROPHIES

Hairs are cylindrical structures made up of modified epithelial tissue. They are divided into four groups; those of the scalp, of the beard, eyebrows or eyelids, and those known as *lanuga*, found on almost every part of the surface of the body. The different shadings of the hair depend on the nature and amount of pigment material found in the hair cells. White hair is destitute of pigment matter. The color of the hair grows darker from infancy to adult life. The amount of elasticity and strength of the hair is truly remarkable. A well-developed hair is said to be able to lift three pounds.

The hair is embedded in the skin in what is known as the hair follicle, a small pear-shaped body, composed of connective tissue fibre, bloodvessels and medullated nerve fibre, and receives its nourishment from the papillæ at its base, the hair bulb being the terminal expansion of the root.

The hair follicle or sac is a flask-shaped sac, enveloping the root of the hair, opening externally by a funnel-shaped mouth. All parts of the hair are subject to disease, as are other parts and organs of the body, confined either to the root, shaft or nutritive supply. There may be complete or partial loss of color, atrophy or hypertrophy from constitutional or local causes, parasitic affections, as seen under the different forms of tinea; also, a partial or even complete alopecia.

CANITIES

This disease may be acquired through disease processes

or heredity. It may come on suddenly or develop by a slow and chronic process. The acquired forms are quite general, occurring early in life, or about the fortieth year, the hair about the temples being the first to change, and gradually the whole head becomes gray or white. The change of color is usually a permanent one. Apart from its loss of pigment, the hair is apparently healthy. Many cases are reported where the hair becomes changed in a single night, due to some great mental shock. Fevers, acute diseases, injuries, prolonged suffering as from neuralgias are favorable factors in producing the disease apart from specific troubles. As a rule, the hair of the beard is not affected until after that of the scalp, and still at a much later date are the hairs of other parts of the body affected by this form of atrophy.

Etiology—Premature canities is generally of hereditary origin, being quite characteristic of some families. Other causes are general ill health, mental or nervous strain, injuries, prolonged dissipation, exhausting diseases, etc.

Pathology—The hair turns gray first at its root, and the loss of color is due to some nutritive change in the hair papillæ, which is probably some form of trophoneurosis.

The treatment is very unsatisfactory, and the prognosis very unfavorable. Study remedies under alopecia.

ALOPECIA

Definition—Abnormal loss of hair due to various causes.

Symptoms—There are four varieties of alopecia, namely: Alopecia senilis, alopecia presenilis, alopecia areata, and alopecia adnata.

Alopecia Senilis—This is loss of hair coming on with the advance of age, which occurs between the age of forty and fifty, and more frequently in men. It is usually preceded for years by canities. It begins usually upon the crown of the head; the hair becoming at first thin, dry, lustreless, and turning gray. The area of baldness spreading symmetrically as the disease advances; the scalp becomes smooth, shiny, sometimes oily.

Pathology—The loss of hair is caused by a gradual atrophy of the skin and subcutaneous tissue from which the hair follicles lose their vitality and also atrophy. The disease, no doubt, begins in the nerve and blood supply, which, owing to the trophic process, is soon cut off.

Prognosis—The loss of the hair is usually permanent.

Treatment—Nothing can be done except to treat the general health of the patient and in that way modify the disease.

Alopecia Presenilis—SYMPTOMS—The form is quite similar to the preceding form, except that it begins earlier in life, between the age of twenty-five and thirty years. It usually begins about the forehead and spreads backwards, though it may begin as the senilic form. Its progress may be rapid, or it may run a slow chronic course.

Pathology—The pathology is very similar to the senile form; simply the atrophic process begins earlier in life.

Etiology—Pathologists tell us that both forms are due to heredity, but that is very indefinite, and comes no nearer to the cause than if the causes had not been mentioned. In our study of its miasmatic causes we find it due wholly to latent syphilis engrafted upon a psoric base.

Treatment—REMEDIES—Sil., Tub., Psor., Ars., Graph., Sulph., Nat. mur., Phos., Cal. c., Cal. sulph., Fluor. ac., Kali carb., Kali phos., Alum., Baryt. carb., Kali iod., Lyc., Mer. viv., Nat. carb., Pet., Sars., Sep., Syph.

Alopecia Areata—(or Circumscripta)—DEFINITION—

Baldness appearing in sharp and well defined patches on the scalp, or other hairy parts of the body.

SYMPTOMS—The hair falls out in a small spot, and the spot or patch increases in size from the periphery; they may be single or multiple, or one or two patches may coalesce, very much increasing the size of the bald spot. The skin of the affected part is usually smooth, pinkish or whitish in color, yet there is no other alteration, although the disease often runs a prolonged chronic course. Sometimes the new growth of hair is finer and often of a lighter color.

Diagnosis—The circumscribed patch, the suddenness of its disappearance, and the normal condition of the surrounding hairs are diagnostic features.

Prognosis—The prognosis is always favorable. The alopecia is only temporary, although some cases are slow and difficult to cure.

Etiology—There is nothing positively known concerning the etiology of the disease, although by many authors it is thought to be a trophoneural affection, and by others a parasitical disease. I am inclined to believe much in the latter cause, as frequently the progress of the disease is stopped at once by a few drops of Acetic acid or alcohol upon the part. Besides, when we consider the progress of the disease, involving a row of hairs, or rather hair bulbs around the central patch, if it was a trophoneurosis, it would not necessarily confine itself to a round or oval patch, or progress the same at all points of the circle. The disease is most frequently met with in children of a tubercular taint, and in Chicago the majority of these cases come from the stockyard district.

Treatment—The remedies most frequently indicated in this disease are those generally employed in the treatment of tonsurans or tinea circinata. This disease should be classified with tinea. The following remedies for consideration and given in the order of their therapeutic value in this disease are: Teuc., Tub., Tellur., Rhus tox., Sepia, Rumex, Sulphur, Psor., Mer. viv.

Alopecia Adnata—Definition—A transient congenital form of alopecia.

Symptoms—The form of alopecia is a congenital form of baldness affecting the whole or part of the head. The hair falls out soon after birth, and is replaced by lanuga. Complete baldness is limited usually to certain parts of the head. However, the disease is only transient; within a few months or a year it is restored, or as soon as the nutrition of the child is corrected.

Etiology—Probably due to error in inervation, or to an imperfect assimilation by the child.

Prognosis—Good.

Treatment—The treatment consists in correcting the general health of the child.

ATROPHY OF THE SKIN

It may be defined as a wasting of the skin, either partial or general. The hair, nails and underlying tissues may also be involved. There are two forms: the degenerative and the simple.

Symptoms—In simple atrophy the skin is pale, thin, dry, shrivelled and sometimes pigmented. There seems to be a diminishing of its constituents. The disease may be primary or secondary; general or local. As a secondary process it follows lupus, favus, syphilis, etc. It may, however, result from traumatism, and often follows the course of cutaneous nerves.

The primary or idiopathic becomes a general disease in what is known as atrophy senilis, or the atrophy of old

age. It involves the different tissues, and sometimes the hair and nails. It may be qualitative, or quantitative, or both.

Symptoms—The skin looks shrivelled, dry, wrinkled, often in folds; very loose and mobile, pale or dark in color with brownish, thickened, epidermis or warty concretions, due to sebaceous and sweat gland changes, besides, there is a general weazening or drying up of the tissues.

Prognosis—Unfavorable.

Treatment—Treatment can only be at the best palliative.

LEUCODERMA

Definition—A disease characterized by the absence of the normal pigment matter of the skin. It may be congenital or acquired. The acquired form is called *vitiligo* In the congenital form the absence of pigment is manifest at birth; when it is complete it is called *albinism*. It sometimes extends to the hair of head or other parts of the body.

Albinism—Besides an absence of pigment in the skin there is also an absence of it in the hair, iris and choroid. Usually the skin is of a pure white, but where the integument is very thin, it is pinkish, as the bloodvessels are seen through its transparency. The hair is fine, silky, white, yellowish or of a golden color. Photophobia is generally present, together with a constant movement of the eyeballs. These patients are frequently tubercular, and they are often neither mentally nor physically strong. The disease in quite prevalent in the dark races. The skin performs all its functions normally. Other than its loss of normal coloring matter it is in a healthy state, as far as can be seen. Where the disease manifests itself in spots, as seen in some individuals, it is called leucoderma, or milk skin. The patches are most frequently met with on the hands, wrists, face, chest, and also on the genital regions.

Vitiligo—Definition—An acquired absence of pigment found in spots or patches, although the margin of these spots shows an increased amount of pigment matter.

Symptoms—The disease is found principally in the tropics and among the colored races. At first the patches are small, but they gradually increase in size. The lanuga and hairs undergo the same changes as the skin, becoming perfectly white. There is a tendency for the spots to coalesce. The disease spreads slowly, taking years to affect large surfaces. There is, as a rule, no impairment in the general health, except it be such mental conditions as would naturally develop from the disfigurement.

Etiology—The causes of vitiligo are unknown. It has been noticed, however, to start from or near an existing mole, or from pressure. It occurs alike in both sexes, seldom before twelve years of age, and generally in the colored races. It is probably some form of trophic neurosis. Alopecia areata has been observed to be frequently associated with it.

Prognosis—Not favorable.

Treatment—No special treatment can be given for any form, although the tubercular diathesis appearing in many cases opens a field for investigation.

PART VIII
CLASSIFICATION—PARASITES

Parasitical diseases in which the human skin, as well as animals is affected; preying as they do upon its delicate and complex structure, causing inflammation, irritations, and great annoyances to the individual in numerous ways, offer a broad and comparatively new field for study and investigation, and while bacteriological research has enlarged and simplified our study of these dieseases as to their etiology and pathogenesis, yet by no means has it taught the general pathologist that every human organism cannot be affected by either class, and especially the vegetable parasite. The secret lies in the fact that the majority of our pathologists are materialists, therefore cannot understand the things that do not develop out of that plain. Their conception of life being false, therefore most naturally, their conception of disease is not true. The cause lies within the individual himself, that power which resists the influences of the infectious and contagious disease from preying upon the organism also resists the inroads of the animal or vegetable parasites.

A parasite is a robber in every sense of the word, or one who lives at the expense of another. The one depending upon the other for life is called a parasite, and the one upon which it is depending is called an autosite. Therefore in order to become subservient to a parasite we must first become an autosite. Now an autosite is not a healthy being by any means. No, that power which should have resisted their attack upon the organism has been destroyed by psora or some other miasm, and the

12

house in which the life force dwelleth is no longer an impregnable fortress. So the usurper enters in and sets up his disease processes therein.

VEGETABLE PARASITES

Tinea

There are four well known forms of the vegetable parasite, they are tinea tonsurans, tinea favosa, tinea barbæ, and tinea circinata. Other forms might be mentioned, but we will confine our study to the above forms.

FAVOSA

DEFINITION—Favosa is a parasitical disease caused by a vegetable fungus, known as achorion schönleinii, entering as its special habitat the hair follicle. It sets up its process, developing in a short time small pea sized, circular, pale yellow or sulphur colored, friable, cup-shaped crusts pierced by hairs and accompanied by itching.

Symptomatology—The scalp is the usual location (although it may attack other parts of the body, even the nails), in which it makes its appearance in the form of the above-described lesions.

These cup-shaped crusts, if removed, show a moist and raw surface; occasionally, in severe cases, pus is found. The itching is more or less severe, and has a peculiar musty odor, resembling musty hay or mice. Alopecia sometimes occurs in neglected chronic cases, but usually the hair reappears when the disease is cured. On examining the hairs they appear dull, having lost their lustre of health, and become dry, brittle, and break or split easily. The disease may extend to the nails, when they become opaque, yellowish, furrowed and brittle.

Pathology—The disease is due, as far as appearance is concerned, to the presence of the spores of the fungi above mentioned.

Diagnosis—The small cup-shaped, sulphur-colored crusts perforated with a hair, together with the peculiar odor, is quite diagnostic. The crusts of eczema are not that color, nor are they of the same consistency, and they lack the odor.

TINEA TONSURANS

SYNONYM—Ring worm of the scalp.

This is a contagious vegetable parasite, due to the trichophyton fungus. The lesions appear in reddish patches, circumscribed or irregular. This circular patch is usually surrounded with a ring of vesicles, occasionally pustules; later on it is covered with scales. The lesions increase rapidly in size from the periphery, usually the extent of the patch being from a dime to that of a silver dollar. The disease is superficial at first, but as it ages the hairs become involved, becoming loose, brittle, easily broken, grayish white, dry and lustreless. The skin of the scalp has a puckered appearance, similar to that of the skin of a bird. The patches are apt to coalesce, and in that way increase the diseased surface; except more or less itching, there are no other symptoms.

Etiology—The disease is due to the trichophyton fungus. It is extremely contagious, and can be conveyed by infected brushes, towels, combs, hats, caps, etc. Men are more liable to it than women.

Diagnosis—Diagnosis is often difficult. Microscopic tests may be sometimes necessary. The broken, bent or twisted, stubby looking hairs are quite characteristic. Dropping a few drops of chloroform on the patch, and allowing it to evaporate, imparts a yellowish or whitish color to the diseased hair, while·the healthy hair is not affected. The disease may be confounded with eczema squamosum, seborrhea, psoriasis capitis and other forms of tinea.

Prognosis—The prognosis is favorable.

TINEA BARBÆ

SYNONYM—Barber's itch.

DEFINITION—(Ring-worm of the beard). A disease of the hair follicles of the face and neck occurring in men.

SYMPTOMS—The lesions are tubercles and pustules appearing in rings or patches that are slightly red and scaly. What is peculiar about these patches is that they show a tendency to heal from their centres, while they continue to extend from their peripheries. The hairs are early affected, becoming brittle and loose. Nodules, pustules, and papules appear upon the skin. There may be slight suppuration present, or it may be absent. When there is much oozing crusts form, giving the lesion some appearance like that of pustular eczema. More or less burning and itching are present, and the disease pursues a slow, stubborn, chronic course, which without treatment would last for years. A microscope usually reveals the parasite.

Diagnosis—The reddened patches with tubercles, or papules and pustules, a tendency to heal from the center, the scanty discharge, the freeness by which the hairs are removed, are all quite diagnostic. Some difficulty may be met with, however, in differentiating it from pustular eczema and tinea sycosis.

Etiology—It is quite contagious, and like all other forms of tinea is of sycotic origin, being a sycotic disease of the hair follicles.

TINEA VERSICOLOR

DEFINITION—Tinea versicolor is a contagious vegetable

parasitic disease of the skin, appearing in an erythematous, scaly patch, occurring anywhere on the body and due to the microsporon furfur.

SYMPTOMS—It differs from tinea sycosis probably only in the location of the disease; at least, it is quite similar to it. Should it spread to the scalp, however, it assumes the form of the tonsurans. It commences as a fawn colored, erythematous patch, slightly elevated. dry and rough to the touch, and from the edges of the lesion, dry, branny scales can be rubbed off. Seldom do the patches exceed from one-half to three-fourths of an inch in diameter. The margins being slightly elevated, they have a ringed appearance. Papules and vesico-papules form on this little circlet, which is covered with fine scales. Itching, tingling, or other sensations are present, and the disease progresses in a slow course, developing on the face, hands, chest and anterior surfaces of the body. The fungi are present in great numbers. In tropical countries the disease is more prevalent, and assumes a severe type. Like most tinea, there is a tendency for the disease to heal from the centre of the patch. It is not a self-limiting disease, however, but requires persistent and careful treatment to cure it.

Diagnosis—There can be no mistaking it for any other disease, except it be eczema squamosum; but the well-defined circles, with their elevated papulo-vesicular border, the tendency to heal in the center, verifies the diagnosis.

Etiology—Is said to be easily transmitted from the lower animals, such as from milking cows, handling of dogs, etc., in very susceptible individuals.

True, the tricophyton is always present; but bacteria proves nothing more than a verification of the form of disease, and that factor is not always a constant one. The miasmatic theory, as to the cause of disease, never would

13

be found wanting if we would but carefully examine into its true nature. In this disease, as in all other forms of tinea, the sycotic element is seen to be present when we fully understand its characteristic primary elements as seen and compared with other diseases; we know it to be the *prima-causa*. A suppression of these diseases by local measures develops the worst forms of disease, even malignancies; rheumatism, of a sub-acute or chronic nature, is very apt to follow sooner or later, a suppression of the disease by local measures.

Treatment—No local treatment is to be thought of for any of these diseases. The homœopathic physician is supposed to know that the disease lies behind the tricophyton; that the bacilla of any disease is simply a physical miscroscopic expression of a subversive force, in which the life force in its predisposed weakness (due to psora) has allowed it to enter, not only the organism, but to influence the action of the life force itself, and having such a positive bond with the life force as to prevent it from throwing off the disease. Therefore, in those diseases that are not self-lasting (as seen in scarlet fever or measles), which are also germ diseases, according to the pathologist, and which are thrown off by a violent reactionary process (fever), we must resort to one of two theories. One, that it is a local disease, due to germs, and the other, that it is a constitutional disease, depending on the predisposition of the patient. If it is a local disease, due to a local cause (germs), then all humanity must in time become affected with it; but this we find not to be true in any disease.

To ignore these truths is to follow the teaching of Virchow and the regular school. To receive them as the truth is to follow the teachings of Hahnemann. It really becomes the trial test of our belief in the miasmatic cause of disease as taught by Hahnemann in his *Organon of Medicine*. The remedies most frequently indicated in the different forms of tinea are: Rhus tox, Sepia, Tub., Teuc., Tellur., Sulphur, Medorrh., Thuja, Mer. viv., Amm. carb., Psor., Pet., Nat. carb., Nat. mur., Ars., Sarsa., Anacard., Bov., Lach., Lyc., Mag. sulph., Nit. ac., Nux jug., Ars., Iod., Vinca min., Viola tric., Lapis alb., Mezer., Olean., Cornus cir.

Rhus tox.—Rheumatic diâthesis, vesicular or pustular forms; yellowish or straw colored vesicles; raw, excoriated surfaces or thick, brownish crusts; intense itching and burning; better by motion; vesicles in clusters size of a small pea.

Sepia—Tinea circinata; brownish or fawn colored vesiculo-papular rings; itching, which changes to burning on scratching. Frequent seat of the disease in flexures of the body, face, hands, and anterior surfaces of the body; worse in the spring of the year; dry, brown, rough, herpetic spots, dry ring-worm in delicate skinned brunettes, who suffer with scanty menses; moles and moth spots in different parts of the body.

Tuberculinum—This remedy was first brought into prominence in the treatment of ring worm by Dr. Burnett, of England. It is indicated in light complected persons with blue eyes, suffering from a tubercular diathesis. It becomes a valuable remedy in ring-worm by virtue of its striking, not only at the ring worm, but at the miasmatic basis. "The fungus is only the guest of the disease," says Burnett. The symptoms are ever changing, takes cold easily, loses flesh while living well, melancholy, despondent, morose; white, bran-like, scales cover the lesion; itching worse undressing, after bathing.

Teucrium—Sycotic patients subject to polypous growths; skin dry, hard, covered with thick white scales; much burning and itching.

Tellurium—Tinea tonsurans and circinatus. Red elevated rings on any part of the body; small, bright red spots covered with scales (fawn colored, Sepia). Minute, grayish colored vesicles on the papillary rings; severe itching day and night; elevated rings of vesiculo-papules, with fine stinging, pricking, itching that disappears by desquamation; eruption worse upon the lower extremities.

Vinca minor—Tinea of the scalp, bad smelling, moist eruptions, hair tangled and matted together; corrosive itching with burning after scratching, worse at night (Sulph.)

Viola tric—Tinea favosa. Scurfs on the head, with unbearable burning; thick crusts that pour out yellow pus, matting the hair; dry sulphur colored crusts; urine turbid, offensive, pustular eruptions.

Arctium lappa—Scalp covered with grayish white crusts, alopecia marked; moist, bad smelling discharges, with suppuration of the axillary gland.

Arsenicum—Dry scaly eruption; crusts when scratched exude thin water, which excoriates; much burning and itching, indicated in pale, thin, irritable people.

Lycopodium—Thick, easily bleeding crusts, oozing fetid moisture; gastric symptoms usually present. Symptoms are worse after scratching by warmth and at four o'clock.

Psorinum—Moist or dry, scaly eruptions, pustules and crusts exuding an offensive discharge; skin and eruptions of a dirty gray color. Intense itching not relieved by scratching; worse from uncovering, from cold and in the winter.

Mezereum—Head covered with thick, leathery crusts; copious exudation of thick yellow pus, or pus oozes out from under thick crusts; thick, white crusts that bleed easily when touched; scratching produces crawling, itching and burning.

Staphisagria—Yellow, moist, offensive, scaly eruption; worse about the ears.

Natrum ars—Squamous eruption and excessive accumulation of thin, white, dry scales which, when removed, the skin looks red and angry. As the scales increase the itching increases; itches worse by warmth and by exercise. Dark complected people with black hair, nose constantly stopped up, with dry crusts in the nose.

ANIMAL PARASITES

Pediculus Capitis (Head Louse)

SYMPTOMS—This form of louse lives exclusively on the scalp, producing in its ravages upon the scalp skin moist patches resembling eczema, pustules, crusts, excoriations, and furuncles. The pruritus is severe, causing the affected one to tear and lacerate the scalp with the nails. They occur in poorly nourished, uncleanly, strumous patients, more frequently in children.

Diagnosis—The diagnosis is more frequently made from the appearance of the whitish, glistening nit or egg found glued firmly and in great numbers to the hair shaft, together with the itching and the secondary lesions.

Treatment—Some of the local remedies are Tobacco, Cocculus Indicus, Staphisagria, Sabadilla, etc.

The **Pediculus Vestimenti,** another form very similar to the head louse, found all over the body, quite often concealed in the creases of the under garments.

Pediculus Pubis, or crab louse, called thus from its peculiar crab shaped form of a yellowish color, producing macules, papules, violent itching without any marked eruption, is somewhat diagnostic of their presence.

Pulex Irritans, the common flea, produces hives or wheals which soon appear after being bitten, leaving behind a hæmorrhagic spot; gives great annoyance to sensitive patients by the intense pruritus induced by their bite.

Pulex Penetrans—A West Indian production, which burrows into the skin, especially that of the feet, even under the nails, producing inflammatory processes, ulceration, etc.

Culex Lectularius—Common bed-bug; produces urticaria of wheals. The itching is very intense, resembling that of urticaria. The presence of the insect is easily recognized by the odor.

SCABIES (Itch)

DEFINITION—A disease due to the burrowing itch mite (acarus scabiei). The itch mite burrows into the skin, forming canals known as caniculi. The secretion produced by their presence is very irritating, giving rise to vesicles, papules, pustules, bullæ, wheals, infiltration, and as secondary lesions, crusts, scratch marks, and furuncles.

Symptomatology—They attack, by preference, the fingers, sides of the fingers, wrists, elbows, axilla, knees, joints, feet. The irritation becomes more marked when the itch mite burrows into the papillary layer of the skin, and when the above-named lesions appear. The itching is a constant, persistent and most annoying symptom, manifesting itself in all degrees of severity, depending much, of course, on the sensitivity of the patient. It is worse at night and when the patient is warm in bed, for then the mite becomes more active when the skin is warm.

Relief is only secured by intense scratching or hard rubbing of the affected part; even then the relief is only temporary. The secondary lesions are, of course, due to intense scratching and irritation of the skin. Boils are apt to follow in strumous or tubercular patients.

Etiology—Simple contact does not often produce it. It is said to require frequent and prolonged contact. More cases appear in children than in adults. No sex, age or condition in life is free from it. Uncleanly people are, of course, more liable. The majority of cases occur between the ages of five and twenty-five. Hahnemann's psoric theory is probably the best explanation as to the cause of this very persistent and stubborn disease. A suppression of the disease and the history that follows its suppression is a sad one, well known to every homœopath. See Hahnemann's Chronic Diseases, Vol. I., also introduction to the Organon.

Treatment—REMEDIES—Sulphur, Sepia, Ars., Carbo veg., Tub., Psor., Carbol. ac., Lyc., Puls., Nat. mur., Mer. sol., Rhus tox., Rumex, Hepar, Sil., Sulph. ac. Also study indications under eczema, tinea, and pruritus. The higher the potency given the better the result. A favorable symptom is to see the disease disappear from the hands first, or in the order it first made its appearance, also by amelioration of the pruritus.

PRURITUS

DEFINITION—A paraesthesia of the skin in the form of intense itching, although it may assume other forms of deranged sensation as tingling, crawling, biting, pricking. All of which create an intense desire to scratch or rub the part. Any number of these sensations may be present at the same time.

SYMPTOMS—It may or may not be accompanied with any local changes in the skin. The disease also may be general or local, and if any lesions are present they are usually secondary, induced by scratching. The disease frequently acquires its name from its location, as pruritus ani, or pruritus vulva. Another, by some authors given special mention is pruritus senilis (a pruritus of old people) where the skin undergoes atrophic changes, causing disturbances and disorders in the tactile corpuscle, inducing an hyperesthetic condition of the endings of the nerve filaments; of course, it is not always due to such changes, but probably to some internal neurotic change, or to blood changes, lymph, bile, etc. Again, the disease may be due to disordered secretion or excretion, to heat, cold, climatic changes in many psoric patients, or it may be produced by foods such as shell fish, oat meal, buckwheat flour, strawberries. In pruritus ani the causes may be many; hæmorrhoids (especially the sycotic form) often cause intense pruritus, driving the patient almost to the verge of insanity or suicide. Other local causes are ascarides, gouty states of the system, uterine or sexual irritation, besides animal and vegetable parasites, clothing, etc., together with diseased conditions, as icterous, hysteria, diabetes mellitus, exanthematous diseases, urticaria, drugs, chemicals, plants. It also occurs from reflexes from the sympathetic system; again, it may be due to changes in the skin itself, eczema, scabies, where marked forms of hyperesthesia are present. No better disease can be selected from the great catalogue of diseases than that of pruritus for our study of psora in some of its most rebellious forms, as seen in the eczema of young children and infants, where the parts are frequently found torn, bleeding and disfigured in the frantic efforts of the little patient to relieve itself of that terrible itching that disturbs it, even to the very centres of the little life, which, if relieved by local measures in one part, it soon manifests itself in ano-

ther, or develops new phenomena that are more dangerous to life and more difficult to combat.

Treatment—All local causes are to be given careful
consideration and removed if possible, not forgetting the
diet and general hygiene of the patient, as well as climate,
vocation, habits, or anything that might prove a hin-
drance to the restoration of the patient's health.

REMEDIES—Gels., Ars., Alum., Carbol. ac., Amm. mur,.
Calc., Carbo veg., Caust., Coff., Borax, Canth., Baryt.
carb., Crotal., Cocc. Ind., Dolich., Kali carb., Sulph.,
Nitr. ac., Sep., Thuja, Zinc., Kali bich., Merc. prot.,
Hepar, Tarant., Hydrocot., Collins., Rhus tox., Rhus
rad., Urtic. ur., Staph., Phos., Sil., Bry., Medorrh., Psor.,
Syph., Tub., Tellu., Mez., Ign., Plat., Puls., Rumex, Nux
v., Agar., Dulc., Arg. n., Calad., Caps., Euphorb., Sabad.,
Mag. carb., Ambr., Lach., Berb., Dros., Petrol., Nat.
mur., Lac can.

Abrotanum—Often follows Hepar; skin flabby, hangs
loose.

Acetic acid—Great dryness of the skin with burning
itching.

Aconite—Dry, hot skin in febrile conditions, with
great restlessness, tingling in fingers and all through the
body, with fine pricking.

Æsculus—Pruritus ani with fullness, heaviness and
sticking in rectum, with backache; formication as of
worms in rectum (Cina, Sab.); crawling as of insects
about the waist.

Agaricus—Itching and burning all over the body; chilblains itch, burn, sting like fine needles. Pruritus ani,
burning, crawling, dryness, fullness, itching, pricking,
stinging, tickling.

Ailanthus—The pruritus of scarlet fever (Bell., Bry.);
claret-colored eruption; miliary rash.

Ammonium carb—Itching, stinging, burning vesicles appear after scratching.

Arsenicum album—Intense burning, itching, painful after scratching; skin rough, dry, scaly, dirty looking, scales fine, white, or grayish white, or bran-like, with itching, burning increased by scratching (relieved, Sulph.); fine, itching, pin-point papules, burning after scratching, relieved by moist heat (Nat. mur); hives or nettle-rash with much burning; herpetic eruptions itch and burn like fire.

Arundo maur—Feeling as of insects crawling over loins and shoulders, sometimes over whole body; eruptions miliary or papular.

Astacus fluv—Nettle rash very severe, with itching in liver troubles.

Belladonna—Skin scarlet, red, smooth, shiny, itching, with heat; scratching produces a pleasant sensation; fine vesicular eruption (Rhus), bright red with dryness, heat, itching.

Bryonia—Pruritus after measles < by heat, better by cool air; dry, papillary itching eruption over the whole body; distressing after measles; cannot sleep for it; intense burning, itching eruption after measles, with much thirst for cold water.

Cactus grand—Very troublesome itching, as of flea-bites, on chest and abdomen; < evening when undressing (Nat. mur., Hep., Rumex, Ars., Psor.)

Caladium—Violent corrosive burning in the skin in small places, > by rubbing; sensation as of a fly on the face.

Calcarea carb—Burning itching eruption < towards morning; child scratches until he screams out; itching vesicles between fingers (Sulph., Rhus, Rumex); eczema with intense itching in young children during teething; itching with moist eruptions.

Cannabis sat—Itching all over the body like thousands of needle points, < at night (Aco., Agar.), < when warm, > uncovering.

Capsicum—Burning in the skin like pepper; formication and biting, creeping as from a fly; stinging, burning itching < in the evening, > by continued motion (Rhus).

Cina—Subjective, fine burning, stinging, in the skin; pruritus ani (Sulph., Sab.); violent itching at night; boring in the nose due to an itching and tickling sensation; biting of nails; minor skin affections in scrofulous children.

Clematis erect—Itching over the whole body; redness and swelling of the skin; burning pain and great heat in skin; discharges acrid, purulent; discharges itching and burning at night; sycotic patients, or eruptions following suppressed gonorrhea.

Cocculus—Burning and itching as from nettles in the skin, < evening and undressing (Nat. mur., Rumex, Hep., Ars.); itching on the chest, tibia, axilla, < during pregnancy, open air, when touched.

Coffea—Skin dry in nervous trouble; itching all over body, changes to burning on being scratched or rubbed (Sulph.); pricking of the skin here and there due to itching, fine points (Opium); rubs the nose, then the face, then some other part; creeping, crawling in different parts, very sensitive, nervous, restless, tosses about; indicated in excessive coffee drinkers, after febrile eruptions and nervous diseases, great wakefulness at night and nervous excitement, reflex itching.

Comocladia dent—Corrosive itching of the head and scalp. Tormenting itching of the nose, or of the whole body, painful burning of the face. Great redness of the skin with violent itching, followed by a yellowish vesication.

Croton tig—Painful burning and itching (Rhus), but

part so sensitive cannot scratch it. Sensation in the skin as if hide-bound. Intense itching followed by painful burning, > by gentle rubbing; itching of scrotum followed by voluptuous sensation; great redness of the skin with vesicles and pustules.

Cubeba—Fiery flush all over the body; fine papular eruption with intense itching.

Dolichos pru—Prurigo. Tettery dry eruption on extremities. Invisible eruption with violent itching, < night, < scratching; during pregnancy. Terrible itching over the whole body, with swelling of the face; compelled to scratch constantly without relief; < warmth of bed, cold bathing, burning after itching ceases, desquamation of small scales.

Dulcamara—Sticking and itching, crawling as of insects; nettle rash with much itching, < warmth > by cold (reverse, Hep.) Burning of the skin when rubbing >. Motion, warmth, gentle scratching.

Euphorbium—Biting, stinging, gnawing, burning itching > motion (Dulc., Rhus). Eruptions on hairy and covered parts, < lying down, or getting near the fire.

Euphrasia—Intense itching of the eyes, eyelids, nose; constant desire to rub hard, bores into the eyes and nose; itching with sneezing; itching intense in the eyes, with weeping; smarting in the eyes after rubbing; itching here and there all over the body at night; burning and formication of the parts. Indicated in hay fever, catarrhal troubles after measles.

Gambogia—Itching and formication in different parts of the body, < at night; after scratching burning. Biting as from ants.

Graphites—Violent itching in eczematous surfaces, eczema rubrum and fissure, < on face, hands, arms, genitals; continued itching, < at night (Sulph.), intense itching and burning followed by oozing of a sticky, viscid fluid; weeping following the itching of a honey-like fluid, or skin dry, hard, leathery-like with deep-seated itching; fissures and bleeding scratch marks after scratching; often no amount of scratching relieves, scratches until the surface weeps or bleeds; < warmth, bed (Sulph.), or a draft of air.

Hepar sulph—Burning, itching, or throbbing; itching like urticaria, being sensitive to touch (Arn., Bell., Lach.); < hands and fingers, < by cold, uncovering.

Ignatia—Great sensitiveness to drafts of air; itching, fine pricking like flea bites; itching in single points which when rubbed disappear to appear some other place; nervous pruritus with twitching of the muscles, gaping, yawning, sighing, with external nervousness.

Kreosotum—Pruritus < towards evening, so severe as to almost drive one wild; on palms of the hands, fingers, bends of joints; > by warmth.

Lac caninum—Itching as of insects on shoulders and neck, also of the sexual organs of women.

Lachesis—Burning itching and formication, paroxysmal; skin extremely sensitive to touch; < on left side, also < after sleep; itching and throbbing, with yellow vesicles following scratching (Rhus, Dol.)

Natrum mur—Itching, stinging, gnawing itching all over the body; marked erythema after scratching; fine, white or colorless vesicles, itch severely, relieved by scratching; scratches until it bleeds (Mez., Ars., Sulph., Psor., Rhus, Tub.); < undressing, yet < by warmth of bed; < 10 A. M., evening when undressing (Rumex).

Psorinum—Burning, biting, itching; itching so intense could tear out the flesh, not > by scratching (> Sulph.); itching stinging as from a burn (Apis); after suppressed itch or eruptions; > by hot application, heat in general, except heat of bed; < between the fingers, about the joints; itching followed by scaling, fine white scales (Ars., Nat. mur.).

Pulsatilla—Burning itching here and there; < on becoming warm; > by motion, walking (Rhus); fine stinging in the skin; mild, gentle, yielding dispositions, especially women; chilly sensations when itching (Pet.), > when the cool air blows over them.

Ranunculus bulb—Extreme itching in herpes; vesicular eruptions; vesicles burn and itch (Ran. scel.).

Rheum—Pruritus ani, in very sycotic children, with green, strong, sour smelling stools; child's body smells sour.

Rhus ven—Violent itching relieved by scratching, vesicular eruption, purulent secretion after scratching.

Rumex—Intense itching with or without an eruption, greatly aggravated on exposure to cold air, undressing or uncovering. Prairie itch, prurigo, urticaria; impetigo contagioso; itching of a pricking or stinging nature.

Sabadilla—Pruritus ani, from ascarides in nervous children. Tingling in the lower extremities; crawling like ants on the skin. Light complected children with a weakened relaxed muscular system who are nervous.

Sepia—Anti-sycotic remedy.

Itching changes to burning when scratching; great itching in the bends of the joints with copper colored or brownish eruptions; dry, tettery eruption. Herpetic eruption that itches intensely; prickling tingling, itching (Tub. Teuc.); urticaria with sticking, itching < in open air; disappears in warm room; acarus itch after Sulphur < in the evening. Pruritus with herpes in dark complected women; any part of the body < about or after menses. Itching of the genitals > by scratching, which is changed to burning (Sulph.), > by hot applications.

Silica—Dry, pale, or white wax-like skin; all symptoms aggravated by cold or uncovering; deep-seated pruritus; tears the skin until it bleeds; > by hot fomentations, < in open air; children who perspire profusely about the head. Pruritus ani with offensive foot sweat. The general symptoms of the remedy to be considered.

Stillingia—Excessive itching of the legs below the knees with no eruption; itching only on exposure of parts to air; > by warmth and of bed; sycotic pruritus.

Stramonium—Itching over the whole body on awaking in the morning; red itching rash breaks out on back after perspiration; burning heat and redness of the skin; stinging and itching like nettles; < by rubbing after scarlet fever or delirium.

Strontium carb—An anti-sycotic remedy; feeling of tension of the skin (Mag. carb.); when pains cease itching begins, and vice versa; moist sycotic eruption that itches and burns.

Zinc—Itching of the skin in bends of joints; itching comes on suddenly in different parts of the body, similar to the itching produced by lice; frequent violent itching at night, causing great restlessness, especially of the feet and lower extremities; itching points with no eruption, crawling and formication in the skin; sudden stinging, pricking, itching in bed, disappears on touching or rubbing; nervous itching.

PART IX

DERMATOLOGICAL THERAPEUTICS

Remedies

ACONITUM NAPELLUS

Skin eruptions following febrile states, exanthematous diseases. Great restlessness, anxiousness and fear of death is a constant symptom of Aconite; children are constantly tossing and changing position.

Objective: Fiery red nettle rash; skin hot, dry, yet the patient may feel chilly.

Subjective: Burning, tingling in fingers and toes, creeping in skin, with drawing pains, with chilliness; great heat in the skin with shivering; chilliness and shuddering; aggravations < night in bed; lying on left side; from getting wet; exposure to dry north wind, < in the open air.

Diseases; Acute catarrhal inflammations, febrile states, dry coughs, croup, convulsions, dentition; fever quick, rapid pulse; dry, hot skin; great anxiousness and general restlessness; peevishness, jerking, twitching and starting in sleep in fevers, moaning; grating of the teeth.

ACETIC ACID

Burning, dry skin, in dentition (Aco.); skin pale waxen (Ars.); warts broad, flat, dry or moist; dropsy after scarlet fever.

Diseases injurious: Nævi, warts, corns, scarlet fever, small-pox, hectic fever, insect bites, hot skin, red spot on left cheeks, drenching night sweats, in tubercular diseases. Follows China.

Temperament bilious motive.

ÆTHUSA CYNAPIUM

Dryness of skin, or dry, burning, red spots; excoriations in flexures and folds of body (Hep.); eruptions, herpetic, tettery, vesicular, < heat, evening; ecchymosis, black and blue spots over the body, wasting, syphilitic children; child drowsy, stupid after vomiting.

AILANTHUS GLAND

Objective—Red, livid rash, < on face, forehead, miliary, irregular, patchy, measly looking rash; disappearing on pressure; reappearing slowly. Bullæ, large, filled with dark blood (Lach., Crotal., Carbo veg).

Petechia, skin harsh, dry, hot (Bell.).

Scarlet rash, < on forehead, neck, chest. (Malignant scarlet fever), purplish rash with stupor, slow to make its appearance (Bry., Ars.).

Accompanying symptoms, apathy, anxiety, delirium violent, high fever, pulse small, rapid (full, bounding, Bell.); Pupils dilated, photophobia, face hot, red (Bell.).

Temperament—Bil. vital.

ALLIUM SATIVUM

Skin sensitive, dry; wilted.
Itching and burning with swelling (Rhus, Apis.)
Herpetic, itching and burning.
Diseases: Stings and bites of insects (Led., Rhus).
Itching, < face, vulva.
Temperament—Bil. lymph.

ALUMINA

Objective—Skin dry, rough, chapped (Graph., Tub.).
Humid crusts on scalp and arms (Mez., Pet.)

14

Bleeding rhagades on hands and forearms; discharges copious, thick, yellowish.

Diseases—Indolent ulcers, chilblains, boils, felons, injuries, lepra, eczema rubrum and fissum, tinea capitis, herpes.

Subjective—Intolerable itching of the whole body; < getting warm in bed; scratches until skin bleeds, then painful; eruption, scabby sore, or dry tetter with formication; < afternoon, evening, every other day; new moon (Sil.); eating potatoes, warmth of bed.

AMBRA GRISEA

Objective—Swelling of the feet; of a gouty nature; dryness of the skin; discharges grayish and salty; suppressed itch or herpes.

Subjective—Burning herpes; tetter on soles of feet; itching papules in beard; raw, sore places in groins and under knees; veins distended and puffed out during the menses. Warts and corns very sore (Arn.).

Diseases—Warts, corns, eczema, scabies, gouty concretions in joints (Borac. ac., Colch., Led., Ars., Mag. m.), < early morning, walking, evening in bed; adapted to lean, aged persons or to young women.

> lying on painful side (Bry).

Temperament—Sang. lymp. nervous.

AMMONIUM CARB

Objective—Boils about ears, nose, on the tip of nose, face, cheeks, corners of mouth, chin, neck. Discharges copious, corrosive, watery; eczema in bends of extremities (Sep., Graph., Pet.); excoriation in groins, on the genitals and anus; freckles; glands of neck affected; purple rash on chest; redness of whole upper part of body like scarlatina (Ailant).

Eruptions like measles; red, ulcerating tubercles about the elbows and neck; ulcers with fetid pus.

Subjective—Burning pimples, pustules and vesicles on the face; burning, itching herpes; burning, shooting, pulling in corns, as if ulcerating; feet sore, as if frozen; sensitive to cold; violent itching; after scratching, burning blisters appear; itching and stinging of the skin keeping her awake; malignant scarlet fever; blood red, miliary rash; putrid sore throat; erysipelas of old people when cerebral symptoms develop.

Diseases—Papules, pustules, burning vesicles, flat ulcers, malignant scarlatina or receding scarlatina; erysipelas of old people, psoriasis; stout women who lead a sedentary life, scrofulous children.

Aggravations—Cold, wet weather, from washing; after rubbing or scratching.

Ameliorations—Lying on abdomen (Acet. ac., Puls.).

Temperament—Sang. lymp.

ANACARDIUM

Objective—Bright scarlet eruptions upon the whole body; herpetic eruptions, painless, pimples with red areola and pus at the tips on the upper arm; intense redness of the skin; eruption of little blisters, with unbearable itching. Chest, neck, axillæ, upper arms, abdomen, scrotum and thighs covered with raised crusts, discharging thick, yellow pus; blisters, discharging a yellow, transparent liquid, hardening to a crust in the open air; effects like those of Rhus tox. on the skin. Erysipelatous swelling of the arms and legs.

Scarlet redness of the skin; syphilitic ulcers, yellowish or a violet color, much swollen and everted; found on the lips, hands, legs, soles of the feet; herpes and ulcers on the scalp, with thick humid crusts.

Subjective—Formication and itching, as of ants; great burning of the skin; burning and stinging herpes; lancinating, burning, deep-seated pain in tumors.

Diseases—Scarlet fever, herpes, dark red erythema, warts on palms of the hands, pemphigus, furuncles, smallpox, adenitis, abscesses, erysipelas, measles, syphilis, scurvy, and pruritus.

Aggravation—Coffee.

ANAGALLIS ARVENSIS

Objective—Skin rough, dry all over; dry bran-like tetter in rings; ulcers and swelling of the joints; sensation on the skin of the forehead as if too tight.

Aggravation—Passive motion and touch.

Used in snake bites and for the expulsion of splinters from the skin (Sil., Hep.).

Diseases: Ringworm (similar to Sep. and Tellur.), ulcers, etc.

ANGUSTURA

Objective—Flat ulcers, eating into the bones; bones of the arm affected.

Subjective—Skin irritable, burns, has to uncover the arms; itching in the evening in bed; tenderness and pain in ulcers.

Aggravation—In bed and after rubbing.

Diseases—Flat ulcers eating into the bone; pruritus, impetigo.

ANTHRACINUM

Objective—Carbuncle, sloughing with abundant ichorous pus, gangrene, felon, small or large epidermal vesicles fill with serum; blisters on the palms of the hands; contents of vesicles contain a yellowish, reddish, or blackish fluid; black or blue blisters; black blisters that are fatal in twenty-four hours; carbuncle with erysipelatous inflammation; phlegmonous or gangrenous erysipelas; umbilicated pustules yellow or blue; hæmorrhagic pustules; blue boils; papules and pustules with great edema; anthrax pustules; deep in the subcutaneous tissue.

Subjective—Skin dry, violent itching and burning (Ars.)

Diseases—Malignant pustule, black vesicles, malignant erysipelas, malignant scarlatina, boils, anthrax, carbuncle; carbuncle with horrible burning pains.

ANTIMONIUM CRUDUM

Objective—Boils in the perineum; pustules like variola; chilblains with redness; horny callosities on the feet, corns; pustules with yellow brown scurf; ulcerating warts; vesicles resembling chicken-pox; skin hard, horny, callous, thick; ulcers deep, flat, fistulous; urticaria with red areola; before small-pox appears great oppression; small-pox and other eruptions with diarrhœa.

Subjective—Violent burning and stinging, with nettle rash.

Diseases—Favus, lichen, eczema, ulcers, small-pox, chicken-pox, warts, corns, callosities, acne.

Aggravation—In damp, cold weather, in the spring; lying down at night, and in a warm room.

Amelioration Cold, open air; sitting up.

Temperament—Sang. vital.

APIS MELLIFICA

Objective—Erysipelas with redness, much edema; edematous swelling of the skin during desquamation; urticaria red, inflamed, edematous; red spots like bee stings; skin has a swollen and bloated appearance; skin hot, red, edematous or pale, waxy, almost transparent; intensely deep red rash; bright red pimples upon the skin; hard, purplish spots upon the skin; hives, red, inflamed, with violent itching and stinging, worse from warmth of bed; better in the open air; urticaria like bee stings, with intolerable itching at night; erysipelas with edematous swelling and burning, stinging pains; measles confluent, with edema; scarlet fever with intense redness, burning and stinging of the skin; painful swallowing, scanty urine; scarlet fever followed by dropsy; inflammations of the brain following suppressed eruptions; carbuncle with burning, stinging pain; ulcers, with much edema.

Subjective—Intolerable itching and burning, stinging like bee stings; burning, stinging, itching, sensitive to touch.

Diseases—Urticaria ulcers with burning, stinging pains, scarlet fever, measles, erysipelas, anthrax, furuncle, herpes, papillary eruption, miliary rash.

Aggravation—From heat, warm room, getting wet.

Amelioration—Open air, bathing with cold water, uncovering, sitting.

Temperament—Sang-lymphatic.

ARGENTUM NITRICUM

Objective—Skin blue, violet or bronze colored, even to black, cyanotic in scarlet fever or small-pox; eczema on the genitals.

Subjective—Burning, itching as from flea bites, or like electric shocks; itching, biting, pricking; indicated in withered, dried-up, old looking, thin, scrawny people.

Aggravation—Cold food, eating sweets.

Amelioration—Open air, desires the cold wind to blow on them, better bathing in cold water.

Temperament—Sang-motor.

ARNICA MONTANA

Objective—Black blisters on the feet; discharges brownish, blood streaked, copious, yellowish, watery or purulent; ulcers after injury; erysipelas after traumatism becoming vesicular or gangrenous; skin cold, blue or black, dry like parchment; peels off in scales, like fish scales, dark red, hot swelling; skin red, hot, edematous after injuries; dark red erythema with small semi-transparent vesicles accompanied with heat, intolerable itching tenderness, and soreness; varicose veins and ulcers; torpid, bluish colored, no pus, but a watery fetid secretion, great soreness and tenderness.

Subjective—Painful soreness and tenderness; skin hot, hard, shining, swollen, much soreness and tenderness; eruptions of all kinds, following injuries, falls, bruises, contusions.

Aggravation—At rest, lying down, from wine, touch (Zinc.); better by motion and gentle contact.

Temperament—Bil-motor.

ARSENICUM ALBUM

Objective—Arsenicum is a deep acting remedy, and produces almost every known lesion upon the skin. Skin dry like parchment; pale, shrivelled, wrinkled, rough, dirty looking; skin cold and blue (Carbo veg.). Skin dry, scaly, bran like, with itching and burning; eruption like fish scales; wax like, dirty, white skin; petechia or ecchymosis following many eruptions in febrile diseases, accompanied with much burning and great·loss of strength; scarlatina eruption delayed or suddenly becomes pale or livid, with petechia; waxy skin in post-scarlatina; small transparent vesicles itching and burning; pustules itch and burn; herpetic eruption with itching and burning; rash goes in suddenly, producing stasis; ulcers with burning pain; discharge watery, greenish yellow, offensive; erysipelas vesicular, gangrenous; swelling of the hands, feet and face, following eruptions; anthrax burns like fire; discharge thin, ichorous, offensive.

Subjective—Burning sensations in all lesions, itching and burning; ulcers burn like fire.

Diseases—Burns, abscesses, eczema, epithelioma, lupus, erysipelas, ecthyma, gangrene, herpes, impetigo, lichen, leprosy, pemphigus, purpura, psoriasis, rupia, itch, malignant ulcers, small-pox, urticaria, malignant scarlet fever, etc.

Aggravation—Lying with the head low after midnight, or from one to two A. M. or P. M. Cold food, cold drink; cold air (Phos.).

Amelioration—Sitting up, heat, hot fomentations.

Temperament—Sang-ment-vit.

ARSENICUM IODIDE

Objective—Chronic, scaly eruptions; dry scaly eruptions, cancer or malignant diseases of the skin, with glandular affections, stony hardness of the glands.

Subjective—Burning, itching, and formication in the eruptions.

ARUM TRIPHYLLUM

Objective—Eruption like scarlet fever, followed by desquamation; eruption all over the body, like scarlet fever; skin peels off afterwards; desquamates in flakes two or three times; face swollen, red; lips and corners of the mouth swollen, sore, cracked and bleeding; putrid sore throat; nose stopped up; glands swollen; child picks at the lips, face or chin until raw, in fevers.

Subjective—Itching, with rapid desquamation after scarlet fever; discharge ichorous, excoriating.

Temperament—Sang-motor.

ASAFŒTIDA

Objective—Dark red, hot swelling of the skin; ulcers with thin, fetid, ichorous, bloody discharges; edges raised, hard, blue; ulcers deep, flat, with fistulous openings; ulcers affecting the bones; ulcers bright red, raw in appearance, covered with tenacious lymph; ulceration from burns or scalds, very sensitive; patient dreads the sore to be touched (Arn.); eruptions flat, painful; ulcers with high, hard, blue edges, sensitive to touch; shooting pains in the ulcer (Hepar, Nit. ac.).

Subjective—Ulcers very sensitive; shooting, itching, pricking, burning in the ulcers.

Diseases—Adenitis; syphilitic ulcers; old scars break open and turn black; fistulous openings, necrosis and caries of the bones; nightly bone pains; antidotes Mercury

Aggravation—After mercury, by contact.

Temperament—Sang-lymph-nervous.

ASTACUS FLUVIATILIS

Objective—Anti-sycotic remedy. Nettle rash all over the body in liver troubles; jaundice of children; thick, crusty eruption on the scalp, with enlarged lymphatic glands.

AURUM METALLICUM

Objective—Dark yellow skin; deep ulcers affecting the bones after the abuse of mercury (Asafœ.). Condylomata; blisters upon the legs of a dingy yellow color; osteo-nodes on the tibia (Mer., Kali iod., Fluoric ac.): dry crusts; deep syphilitic ulcers, bluish in color, with fistulous openings (Asafœ.); caries of the bones of the lower extremities; ulceration of the bones of the nose; people of despondent, melancholy, suicidal tendency.

Aggravation—From mercury, in the morning; in winter and in open air; better by warmth and by moving.

BAPTISIA TINCTORIA

Objective—Eruptions like measles or urticaria; foul, gangrenous, eating syphilitic sores; confluent small-pox, with tardy eruption; petechia in typhoid fever or rose colored spots.

Subjective—Burning all over the body, worse on the face; face dark, dusky looking in fevers.

Temperament—Bil-motor-temp.

BARYTA CARBONICA

Objective—Red, excoriated, moist, burning places between the scrotum and thighs; skin does not heal readily; dry exanthemata; excoriation and oozing; swelling and induration of the glands; scrofulous, dwarfy children, who do not grow. Great sensitiveness to cold; offensive foot sweats; toes, heels become sore from perspiration (Sil.).

Subjective—Intolerable tingling over the whole body, itching, pricking, burning, here and there, not relieved by scratching.

Aggravation—Washing the affected part, when thinking about his disease.

Temperament—Sang-lymp.

BELLADONNA

Objective—Skin dry, hot, smooth, shiny, tense, swollen; hot to touch; extreme redness with or without rash; scarlet fever, red, smooth, skin over the whole body; erysipelas, skin bright red, swollen, smooth, shiny; red spots with vesicles; all eruptions sensitive to touch.

Subjective—Skin painfully sensitive to contact (Am. c.); high fever, face red, flushed; pulse full, rapid; drowsy; sleepy or with delirium; great dryness and heat of the skin; creeping, crawling, itching or pricking, darting and biting.

Diseases—Anthrax, boils, chilblains, erysipelas, inflammation, acute erythema, herpes facialis, measles, scarlet fever, nettle rash, itching or pain appears and disappears suddenly.

Complementary to Calcarea carb.

Aggravation—From touch, motion, noise, cold air, bright light, while drinking, uncovering the head.

Amelioration—Rest, standing or sitting; warm room.

Complications—Delirium, coma, convulsions; complications of internal organs.

BENZOIC ACID

Gouty or rheumatic diathesis in the tertiary stage of sycosis (Borac. ac., Colch., Lith. carb., Thuja, Ledum).

Objective—Gouty concretions in the joints, more especially the small joints, fingers and toes. It follows Colchicum frequently in gouty states. Nodosities and concretions can be felt under the skin; strong scented beer colored urine; warts round, sessile and thickly grouped together.

Subjective—Pains in joints of right great toe, < at night; abundant gouty concretions about the joint; eruption of red spots on the fingers; intense itching in palm of right hand; itching after scratching leaves an agreeable sensation followed by burning.

Diseases—Gouty concretions, warts, red moles, acne; papules large, red, sore, tender to touch.

Aggravation—Wine drinking (Zinc.), night, pressure, heat.

Temperament—Sang-motor.

BERBERIS VULGARIS

Objective—Anti-sycotic. Blotches like nettle rash on upper arm; yellow spots on the abdomen (Lyc., Sep., brown); herpes around the anus; clusters of red pimples with a reddish areola, tips contain pus. Pea-shaped vesicles on lower lip (Rhus, Nat. mur.); warts on eyelids; warts small, fine, thickly grouped together all over the trunk of the body, with small thread-like attachments; filiform warts (second stage, sycosis).

Subjective—Biting, pricking, burning, itching in the skin with increased warmth (a sensation); red spots on the skin feeling like a mosquito bite; burning and pricking along the edges of the hair; follows Arnica, Bry., Kali bich., Rhus tox.

Diseases—Gouty complaints; lithic diathesis; renal and vesical symptoms predominate.

Aggravation—Motion, jarring, riding in a carriage.

Temperament—Bil-ment-motor.

BISMUTH

Objective—Ulcers gangrenous, bluish parchment-like; itch like eruptions; eruptions following or developing from gastric symptoms.

Subjective—Corrosive itching on side of tibia; external dry, burning heat.

Diseases—Dry, gangrene (Secale); ulcers bluish, gangrenous; often used locally on ulcers.

Aggravation—Touch; cold bathing in many cases.

BORAX

Objective—Eczema of scalp and face in young children and infants; intertrigo between the thighs in young infants (Hep.); slightest injury suppurates (Hep.); Red papules on the cheeks and around the chin; dry, hard, callous spots on feet and hands (Graph., Sil.); wilted, wrinkled skin (Ars.); in children with aphthæ. Hair tangles, breaks and splits easily.

Subjective—Fear of falling; sensation of a cobweb on the face.

Severe itching about finger joints, must scratch violently. Borax follows Cal. carb., Phos., Sulph., Sanic, and is incompatible with Acetic acid.

Diseases—Erythema and intertrigo of children; eczema of face and scalp; erysipelatous inflammation; matting of the hair; aphthous sore mouth; child screams before passing urine.

Aggravation—Downward motion; damp, cold weather; before urinating.

Amelioration—Pressure, holding tightly.

Temperament—Sang-vit-lymph.

BOVISTA

Objective—Tettery eruptions, dry or moist; sweat in axilla smells like onions; awkward people, who drop things easily (Apis); urticaria covering the whole body. Blotches one or two inches in diameter.

Rash, pimples with burning itch; moist or dry herpes. Warts and corns with shooting pains (Nit. ac.). Red, scabby eruptions on thighs and bends of knees; comes on during hot weather and at full moon; urticaria with rheumatic lameness (Rhus, Dulc.).

Subjective—Itching on getting warm (Sulph.); continues after scratching; shooting pains in warts and corns, rash and pimples, with burning itching. Intolerable itching at tip of coccyx, scratches until parts become raw.

Diseases—Warts, corns, eczema, urticaria, tubercles, red pimples; eruptions following painful menstruation; aggravation < in the evening.

Bovista is an antidote to the bad effects of tar applied locally in skin diseases. Follows Rhus tox. in chronic urticaria.

Temperament—Sang-lymphatic.

BROMIUM

Objective—Indicated in people with light blue eyes, flaxen hair, fair, delicate skinned, scrofulous girls; swellings of the glands, with stony hardness (Iod., Iod. ars., Con., Hep., Tub.). Ulcers with smooth edges; discharges watery, excoriating; cancer of mammæ; swelling of the glands after scarlet fever.

Sensation of weakness and exhaustion in the chest. Boils on arms and face; eczema capitis, with profuse oozing of a dirty colored, bad smelling discharge; scalp covered as with a cap of crust (Hep., Mez.). Thin, white, delicate skinned girls.

Subjective—Scalp tender. Internal burning heat in skin, after chill. Tickling, itching, pinching, or stitches in the skin.

Diseases—Boils, pimples, cancer of breast or glands, eczema, moist herpes.

Aggravation—Evening.

Temperament—Sang-lymphatic.

BRYONIA

Objective—Eczema in bends of extremities (Graph., Sep., Pet., Psor.); eruptions come forth slowly in scarlet fever and measles. Hard, inflamed, shining swelling of the part affected. Skin yellow or saffron colored in icterous, cutaneous eruptions, usually dry. Dry, itching eruption over the whole body; erysipelatous eruptions; secondary affections of lungs, heart and different organs, following suppressed eruptions, pleuritis, pneumonia, variola with dropsy; rheumatic diathesis; dark haired and dark complected people, who are cross and irritable when sick, and usually constipated.

Subjective—Aching soreness during eruptions. Burning

itching. Gnawing itching and pain; pricking, darting pains in corns. Tearing, drawing pains, < motion. Cold feeling in ulcers. Purpura rheumatica.

Diseases—Exanthematous eruptions, boils, pimples, acne, ulcers, arthritic nodes, nettle rash, chilblains, lichen miliaria, purpura rheumatica, petechia, erysipelas of the joints.

Skin white or red streaked in inflammations, radiating red streaks.

Aggravation—Heat, morning, motion; suppressed eruption.

Amelioration—Quiet, rest, lying down, cool bathing, light pressure.

Temperament—Bil-motive.

BUFO

Objective—Red, purplish streaks on the neck or other parts. Skin greenish, oily or dirty yellow. Tetter, and eruptions of small nodules. Phlyctenoid eruption, discharging a thin, yellowish fluid. Black, or bluish swelling about the thumb nail. Malignant pustule. Carbuncles with blue areola extending far around (Carbo veg., Anth.).

Subjective—Skin diseases in patients suffering from epilepsy. Yellow blisters on soles of feet and palms of hands, burn severely. Stitches in the skin preventing sleep. Ulcers with burning pains (Ars.).

Diseases—Carbuncles, anthrax, ulcers, boils, papules, chilblains, erysipelas, malignant pustules, eczema, pemphigus.

CALADIUM

Objective—Eczema of the genitals, mosquito and insect bites, burn and itch intensely (Led.). Rash with white vesicles on the wrist and forearm; red pimples, itch and burn; white, suppurating pimples with red areola; painful pimples on septum of nose; suppressed urticaria followed by oppression of the chest or dyspnea.

Subjective—Violent corrosive itching; must touch the parts, but cannot scratch them (Coff.). Frequent attacks of violent corrosive burning in small spots on the nose, cheeks, toes, fingers and other places; rubs them gently, but cannot scratch, as it greatly increases the suffering. Pruritus vaginæ; inducing onanism (Zinc). Sweat attracts the flies.

Diseases—Pustules, papules, urticaria, eczema of the genitals, pruritus of the vagina, voluptuous itching in genitals, troublesome eruption following pruritus.

Aggravation—Motion (Bry.), evening scratching.

Amelioration—From perspiration, touch and gentle rubbing, quiet, daytime. Complementary to Nit. ac.

Temperament—Phlegmatic.

CACTUS GRANDIFLORUS

Objective—Dry, scaly herpes, about the joints, no itching. Cactus is an anti-sycotic remedy.

Subjective—Sensation of constriction about different parts of the body. Pruritus ani, feeling as if rectum was swollen (Aloe); pricking in as from pins. Skin edematous, pale, very white, especially in the feet in heart diseases. Troublesome itching, as from flea bites on chest and abdomen; itching disappears in the evening.

Diseases—Herpes dry, scaly, do not itch; anasarca of the skin. Purpura, with hæmorrhages from internal organs.

Temperament—Nervo-bilious.

CALCAREA CARB

Objective—Leucophlegmatic, blonde hair, light complexion, fair skin, soft flabby muscled women with pale, white skin; weak, timid, easily exhausted, walking, or ascending a height. People who perspire easily; take cold easily; exhaust easily. Eczema, thick, moist or dry crusts on the face and scalp; eruptions vesicular all over, sometimes inflamed; scald head, thick crusts with yellow pus (Hep.). Lips chapped and cracked and corners of the mouth ulcerated (Nat. mur., Nit. ac., Tub., Pet.); very small warts in bunches on the lower lip. Ulcers inside of lower lip, light yellow surrounded by redness, painful on contact with tongue; varicose veins with burning in the veins. Cancer of the breast, very sensitive and painful to touch. Chaps and rhagades from working in water (Graph., Tub.); elevated red stripes on the tibia, with severe itching and burning. Chronic forms of urticaria, disappearing in cold air; miliary eruption over the body, especially abdomen; itches so that child scratches until it screams; follows Belladonna after scarlatina in leucophlegmatic temperaments. Fresh leprous spots on the chin; milk white spots on the skin; skin eruptions covered with bran-like scales (Syph., Ars., Psor.). Herpes burning. Ringworm with scaly skin; eruptions with thick scales and yellow pus under them; pustular eruptions on head, neck, shoulders and buttocks. Acne indurata or punctata, with oily appearance of the face or perspiration of the face appearing in large drops (Mer., Sil.); eczema of the scalp with enlarged cervical glands in fleshy, scrofulous children who are self-willed, and perspire profusely about face and head. Small vesicles resembling the itch on hands and fingers with moist, sweaty palms (Sil.). Calcarea eradicates the predisposition to boils, boils of neck, shoulders, arms; ulcers with a red, hard, swollen circumference, feeble granulations, usually painless, discharging

15

yellowish pus; encysted tumors; hard swellings; warts, round, soft at base, almost natural color of skin, upper surface hard and tough, whitish, horny. Warts appear, bleed and disappear, or suppurate and form ulcers; ulcerating warts. Warts inflamed with stinging, finally suppurating. Small wounds suppurate and do not heal (Hep.). Fallng out of hair from squamæ of head.

Itching, < towards evening and in bed; eruptions, burn and itch; stinging, burning itch with heat, pricking, smarting, itching, < by cold, yet not > by heat; icy coldness of head and feet; crawling and itching in arms; tubercles or labia with stinging, burning and itching.

Aggravation—Morning and evening; warmth. motion, standing, touch.

Amelioration—Rest, dry weather; summer, fresh air; rubbing or scratching. Complementary to Bell.

Diseases—Adenitis, boils, corns, warts, dandruff, encysted tumors, eczema capitis or facialis; freckles, herpes, measles, urticaria, psoriasis, prurigo, pruritus, pemphigus, rhagades, after scarlatina, ulcers, varicose veins, cancer of breast, vesicles, pustular eruptions, tubercular skin diseases of all forms. Children are usually deficient in bone and excessive in the development of flesh, which is never firm or hard, always pale and flabby.

Temperament—Sang-vit-lymphatic.

CALCAREA PHOS

Objective—Acne rosacea; red vesicles filled with yellow lymph; carious ulcers; eczema with anæmia; dry crusty affections; fistulous or scrofulous ulcers (Cal. c., Sil.); skin diseases, scurfy and scabby in anæmic scrofulous people; skin dark, brownish or yellowish.

Tubercles in the skin. Flabby, shrunken, emaciated children, whose bones do not develop well; rachitis in children (Cal. Sil., Sulph.); exostosis of the extremities, dark complected, anæmic patients (reverse, Cal. c.), with weak spines and curvature of the bones.

Subjective—Burning itching and formication of the skin, < damp weather; itching and burning as from nettles; itching and biting in small places, long before they show any lesions. Complementary to Ruta.

Aggravation—Exposure to dampness, cold, changeable weather.

> summer; dry weather.

Temperament—Bil-motor.

CALCAREA SULPH

Objective—Scarlet rash, scarlatina, with swelling of the soft palate; suppurating pustules and nodules; isolated pustules; pustules on hands, fingers, about the margins of the nails, yellowish in color, flat and with scanty, yellowish discharge; skin affection with greenish, brownish or yellowish crusts. Abscesses, boils, carbuncles, papules, controls the formation of pus (Hep., Sil.). Burns and scalds suppurate profusely (Hep.). Suppuration on the hands, fingers or any part following bruises or contusions (Arn., Sulph. ac.). Its sphere of action is in the connective tissue, controlling suppuration (Sil.). Discharges in coughs, gonorrhea, injuries, leucorrhea; yellowish, thick, sometimes lumpy. Blisters on lower lip suppurate, ooze bloody matter; also, on the chin; scabs on the corners of the mouth; ulcers discharge a thick, yellow matter; chilblains suppurate.

Subjective—Itching on soles of feet; pain in ulcers or pustules.

Aggravation—Walking, motion, touch.

Amelioration—Lying down.

Temperament—Bil-motor.

CALENDULA

Objective—Wounds raw and inflamed; old, neglected wounds, or ulcers, become offensive; ulcers, weak, indolent, irritable, inflamed, sloughing, varicose or hæmorrhagic; excessive secretion of brownish yellow pus; sores painful as if beaten (Arn.). Abscesses follow operations; wounds become raw, and inflamed and suppurate; are painful in the morning, as if beaten. Profuse, bad colored, stinking suppuration; articular and clean cut surgical wounds; lacerated or torn wounds; severe injuries of soft parts; it prevents rapid granulation; traumatic affections to secure union by first intention.

Subjective—Most symptoms appear with a chill; stinging pain in wound during the fever; wound painful in the morning; painful, as if beaten, with stinging and throbbing in ulcers. Itching, burning soreness.

Aggavation—Night, evening.

Amelioration—From perspiration, after sleep. (Complementary to Hypericum.)

Diseases—Fresh cuts, wounds, old ulcers become unhealthy. Indolent ulcers. Erysipelas after injuries, for surgical operations; soft warts. Abscesses following surgical operations.

Temperament—Bil-motor.

CAMPHORA

Objective—Erysipelas of face. Erythema from exposure to sun's rays.

Skin cold, bluish, in cholera, or pale and withered; surface cold, yet cannot bear to be covered. Sudden and complete prostration of the whole organism, with great coldness of the surface of the skin. Cholera, dysentery, measles, scarlet fever, small-pox; skin tense, hot, dry, like parchment; petechia over whole body. Scarlet fever with cold, blue hippocratic face; hot sweat on forehead; breath hot, yet child will not be covered.

Sudden sinking away of variola pustules. Skin cold as marble, yet wishes to be uncovered. Cyanosis, external parts turn black.

Subjective—Burning pain when touched.

Aggravation—Cold; cold air, evening, in bed.

Amelioration—From warmth, warm air. Camphor antidotes the majority of the vegetable remedies; it also is the most powerful agent to suppress eruptions or discharges we have at our command. The majority of our mammary abscesses are caused by suppression of the flow of milk by applying Camphor locally.

CANNABIS SATIVA

Objective—Acne rosacea, large nodosities surrounded by red swelling on the nose. Bright red spots on the prepuce.

Subjective—Unendurable fine stitching over the whole body, like a thousand needle points, at night; when perspiring, > uncovering; numb feeling in tips of fingers.

Aggravation—Forenoon.

Temperament—San-ment-nervous.

CANTHARIS

Objective—Erythema from burns, from sun's rays, from the effects of cold; eczema. Gangrene of external parts.

Erythematous inflammation with blebs, bullæ, vesicles, petechia; exudation of yellow serum, copious, raising the epidermis; erythema with ulceration. Burns of first and second degree, with bladder and renal irritation, strangulation and vesicle tenesmus. Vesicular erysipelas, ulceration and gangrene after exanthematous diseases. Variola with dysuria, pemphigus.

Subjective—External burning and smarting. Burning. pricking, stinging, smarting. Painful vesicles or erythema after burns. Ulcers, itching, or tearing pains. Burning and smarting, < when touched; vesicular and erythematous eruptions; burn like fire; to rest in any position. Burning pains in skin with straining to urinate.

Aggravation—When touched.

Antidoted with a high potency and weak solution of alcohol and water locally.

Temperament—Bil-vital.

CAPSICUM

Objective—Fissures and ulceration of the lips (Graph., Pet., Kali iod., Tub.); red dots in the face, and herpes on the forehead, with biting and itching. Skin bloated, flabby (Calc., Apis); acne rosacea, scarlet eruption on neck and breast. Face, extreme redness or with a mapped appearance. Herpes on the face with itching and burning, indicated in light haired, blue eyed, lax fibre and muscle, with a sycotic and psoric basis; always chilly.

Subjective—Burning in the skin as if sprinkled with pepper. Formication, creeping in the skin; corrosive itching, especially in herpes; stinging, burning itching in scarlet fever or measles; itching < from scratching; after scratching soreness and smarting, yet must rub it; skin eruptions, following suppressed gonorrhea.

Diseases—Gonorrhea and eruptions developing from its suppression. Burning herpes, scarlet fever, measles, warts. Pains, constricting burning.

Aggravation—Touch, rubbing, scratching; evening.

Amelioration—Walking; constant motion.

Complications—Brain symptoms, in acute febrile diseases.

Temperament—Sang-lymphatic.

CARBO VEGETABILIS

External parts grow black (gangrene); exhausting diseases, hæmorrhages from mucous outlets, or into the skin; the blood oozes from the relaxed and weakened tissues; cold, clammy sweat after hæmorrhages; venous congestions, cadaverous smelling odors from discharges, skin dry, brittle, in severe fevers; cyanosis of the skin often general in heart troubles. Fine, moist, burning rash; hoarseness following measles; scarlatina, last stage, with cold perspiration; skin turns blue, with sloughing. Leprosy, brownish, red spots. Purpura, all forms; asthenic, small-pox; eruption blue or black; odor offensive; perspiration and coldness of the surface; ulcers, varicose, livid, blue, black, fetid, bleeding easily; burning after bleeding; all discharges offensive (Asaf.); sepsis, sunken features, sallow complexion; hectic, typhoid symptoms, or symptoms of collapse.

Subjective—Burning pains; hæmorrhages, with soreness; ulcers with burning pains.

Diseases—All forms of acute malignancies, fevers, ulcers, carbuncles, boils, sepsis, anthrax, exanthematous diseases, malignant diseases, gangrene, caries, phlegmonous erysipelas, cyanosis. Bad effects of shock in surgical operations. Purpura, small-pox, varicose ulcers, burns, chilblains, gunshot wounds, intertrigo, prurigo, scald head.

Aggravation.—Motion, fat foods, warm room or warm air; evening, in bed.

Amelioration.—Rest, fanning, eructations.

Temperament—Bil-motor.

CARBOLIC ACID

Objective—Severe forms of erysipelas; malignant scarlatina, pustular and vesicular eruptions, sloughing wounds and chronic ulcers; eruption, miliary, over whole body; erythema with vesication, ulceration and sloughing, confluent variola; ulcers with sloughing and foul odor (Carbo veg., Asaf.). Extensive burns and scalds, chilblains that ulcerate; warts that ulcerate; burns that ulcerate, with ichorous discharges. Putrid discharges from all mucous orifices of the body; cancer discharging a dark green, olive fluid; or discharges dark green, copious, acrid, fetid.

Subjective—Pains ulcerative, severe; come suddenly and disappear suddenly (Bell.); numbness of the skin, smarting, burning, tingling; pain, eating, gnawing; comes and goes suddenly. The acid applied to warts does not cease its destructive action, but continues until antidoted (like Ars.).

Diseases—Acne, eczema, impetigo, scabies, psoriasis, leprosy, prurigo, pityriasis, lupus, carbuncles, cancer, sloughing wounds, chronic ulcers, erysipelas, burns and scalds.

Aggravation.—Touch.

Amelioration—Rest.

Antidotes—Cider vinegar, dilute, or glycerine locally; internally, a high potency of Carbolic acid.

Temperament—Nervo-bil.

CAUSTICUM

Objective—Burns; vesicles under prepuce, changing to ulcers. Phagedenic chancre, with jerking pain, watery, greenish, corroding discharge. Chancre with fungus excrescences, yellowish looking skin, more so about the temples; eruptions similar to the blisters from burns; chronic urticaria, appearing more fully in the fresh air. Pemphigus. Itching blotches, burning like nettle rash; eczema pustulosum. Large, jagged, non-pedunculated warts, appearing on any part of the body, even on eye-lids. Injuries heal then break open again; especially is this seen in old scars. Varicose and fistulous ulcers. Phagedenic ulcers. Ulcers bleeding, with vesicles surrounding them; burning in the edges; discharge bloody, corroding, green-ish or grayish. Tubercular ulceration of the skin, chorea, paralysis, epilepsy, following injuries or bruises. Dark haired people with rigid fibre (Nit. ac.); sallow com-plected people.

Subjective—Rheumatic affections with contractions of the muscles. Child wishes to be carried (Ars., Cham.). Itching over whole body. Burning after scratching. Gnawing itching, or complete loss of sensation or motion.

Aggravation—In clear, fine weather, evening; coming into a warm room; bathing, during perspiration.

Amelioration—During wet weather.

Diseases—Burns; blisters on feet; encysted tumors; felons. Herpes on ring finger; nettle rash, nodosities. Tubercles. Warts pedunculated and non-pedunculated, varices, zona, ulcers, eczema, intertrigo in teething children.

Temperament—Lymphatic.

CHELIDONIUM MAJOR

Objective—Sallow, jaundiced complexion; or skin cold and dry; wilted, yellowish gray in liver affections. Acute jaundice with intense itching of the skin. Bright red, lentil-sized, round spots on the face on awakening in the morning. Red, painful papules in different parts of the body. Red, miliary eruption on neck, chest and arms. Crusts exuding moisture and scaling off. Old, putrid smelling ulcers. Eruptive diseases, appearing reflexly from liver troubles. Skin hot with sour smelling sweat. Light complected blondes, subject to gastric and hepatic troubles.

Subjective—Burning pains in skin with stinging, preceding measles (Apis); or like nettles (Urtica urens). Burning spots on the forearm. Intense itching of whole body in ichthyosis, followed by redness and burning. Skin feels cool.

Aggravation—Morning, motion.

Temperament—Bil-motor.

CHAMOMILLA

Objective—Skin moist and burning hot in teething children. Miliary exanthema; red rash on cheeks and forehead; measles, herpes, pimples; vesicles on the face, excoriations in the flexures of the body in children; rash of infants, erysipelas of face, many skin eruptions confined to the face of infants; urticaria in cross, peevish, fretful children; red rash consisting of papules crowded into a small spot. Ulcers sensitive, with inflamed edges. Rhagades of the skin; skin yellow; child looks old, sallow, is cross, irritable, so cross can't live with them scarcely.

Subjective—Burning smartness in the skin. Itching with shuddering in the skin; skin over-sensitive in children; suppurates easily. Burning, smarting, lancinating pain in ulcers, > by cold. Itching worse on perspiring parts. Itching pimples around an ulcer (Hep.). Light brown hair; nervous temperament.

Aggravation—Evening and night, after scarlet fever; during the menses, pregnancy, perspiration, especially after suppressed perspiration.

Amelioration—From warmth while perspiring.

Temperament—Sang-mot-vital.

CHINA OFFICINALIS

Objective—Bleeding after scratching. Boils on the chest. Erysipelatous swelling of the whole body. Nettle rash coming out after scratchig. Skin dry, flaccid, painful sensitiveness of skin; waxy pale or yellow; sweat parboils the skin. Ulcers flat, shallow, with copious discharge; small-pox, (pustules black); hæmorrhage, with great exhaustion; psoriasis, ichthyosis, pemphigus. People who are very sensitive to pain (Coff.); acne following onanism (Nux). Hæmorrhages from all orifices of the body, painless, profuse, exhausting, followed by ringing in the ears and vertigo (Ferrum).

Subjective—Biting itching; boring itching; stinging itching in wounds. Painful sensitiveness in the skin, even palms of hands. Beating in ulcers. Itching in parts lain on. Desire to uncover, but chilly when uncovered.

Aggravation—Night, every other day; slightest touch, draft of air, after scratching, mental emotions, loss of fluids of the body.

Amelioration—Hard pressure.

Temperament—Bil-motor.

CHININUM SULPH

Objective—Urticaria over whole body. from over doses. Red rash over whole body, with severe stinging followed by desquamation. Cancerous ulcers, with thick, livid humid crusts, which later on become dry and black. Sudamina in continued fevers, with red spots. Skin flaccid and sensitive to touch (China, Am. carb., Bell., Lach.). Gangrenous ulcers.

Subjective—Sensitiveness and tightness of the scalp; soreness of the roots of the hair; stinging in eruptions followed by desquamation. Confluent small-pox with hæmorrhage. Suits weakly, florid, sanguine, hæmorrhagic constitutions.

Aggravation.—Touch; change of weather.

Antidotes suppressed eruptions in high potency.
Temperament—Bil-motor.

CHIMAPHILA UMBELLATA

Objective—Scrofula, with indolent ulcers. Tumors of
the mammæ. Glandular enlargements, especially lymphatic. Malignant ulcers, discharging yellowilsh ichor.
Crawling and stinging in ulcer. Cachectic individuals,
broken down in health. Lumps in left breast break into
a small, irregular ulcer, with ragged edges, sloughing
and discharging fetid pus. It is an anti-syphilitic remedy.

CHROMIC ACID

This remedy has been found useful in the bites of
rabid animals, poisoned wounds, phagedenic ulcers.
Symptoms similar to secondary syphilis have developed
from the proving. It is one of the principal ingredients
in corn and wart ointments, which often cause their
disappearance when applied locally.

CHLORAL HYDRATE

Objective—Face pale, bloated, dirty yellow, cadaverous color. Ash-colored face (Plumb.); dry, yellow,
shrivelled. Malignant pustules and carbuncles. Typhoid
states in measles, variola, typhus, typhoid, etc.

Subjective—Stinging and biting here and there as of
insects. Skin extremely sensitive. Bright red or bluish
erythema over the whole body. Pruritus of the whole
skin and mucous outlets. Sensation as of a hair on the
nose.

CICUTA VIROSA

Objective—Purulent eruptions; yellow scurf on the
chin. Impetigo contagiosa. Honey-like crusts on the

face and chin. Eczema of the face; sulphur-colored, soft, friable crusts. Humid, scabby herpes; dark red macules soon form into vesicles finally into pustules, often coalescing. Ashy paleness of the face in children, with convulsions, due to worms or epilepsy. Acne rosacea. Eczema with no itching; exudation dries into a hard, lemon-colored crust.

Subjective—Red vesicles, painful to touch. Herpes or impetigo, with burning and itching.

Temperament—Sang-ment-vital.

CINNABARIS

Objective—Sycotic and syphilitic diseases; suppressed eruptions; condylomati; large cockscomb shaped; red, bleeding easily; large vegetations that bleed easily; warts bleed easily. Warts about the sexual organs bleed profusely (Nit. ac.). Small, shining, red points on the glans penis. Syphilitic phymosis; syphilitic disease of the skin engrafted on a sycotic basis. Ulcers with elevated edges and a discharge of thin, yellowish-green pus. Honeycombed ulcers, with fistulous openings. Sanguine temperament; scrofulous or syphilitic patients.

Subjective—Violent itching of the corona glandis; usually the remedy is free from itching; pains shooting, drawing, tearing, < at night. Burning and itching in some eruptions.

Aggravation—After scratching.

Temperament—Sang-phlegmatic.

CISTUS CANADENSIS

Objective—Vesicular erysipelas, adenitis, herpes on the ear, lupus of the face, mercurial and syphilitic ulcers. Caries of the lower jaw, with suppuration of the glands of the neck. Open, bleeding cancer of the lower lip. Cancer of the breast; hard, thick places on the hands of workmen, with deep, oblique fissures. Tetter on the hands; blisters, oozing after scratching, with swelling and hot feeling. Hip disease with fistulous openings, accompanied with night sweats. Small, painful pimples, that bleed easily. Eruptions on the back like zoster; lupus of the face, with glandular enlargement.

Subjective—Itching all over the body without eruption. Sensation of ants running through the whole body, especially at night. Itching in the ears intense, deep in; crawling itching in throat; eczema with intolerable itching with the formation of thick crusts. Cold feeling or burning in the nose in lupus.

Temperament—Sang-ment-vital.

CLEMATIS ERECTA

Objective—Skin inflamed, red, burning; eruption of blisters, which burst and form ulcers. Eruption of vesicles and pustules; from the vesicles a clear water exudes, and from the pustules a purulent secretion, followed by a formation of scales and crusts. Sometimes this extends over the whole body, always exuding, and accompanied with intolerable itching. Chronic herpes. Eruptions inflamed during the increase of the moon, and dry during the disease, < washing in cold water, warmth of bed, wet applications, if warm. Head and face a solid mass of scabs, dark, rough, adhering firmly, exuding a yellowish fluid; excoriating, healthy skin where it passes over. Chronic, red, humid herpes, with intolerable itching in warmth of bed (Sulph.), and after washing; tendency to rupture, with ulceration of the vesicles. Dark, burning, miliary eruptions, with violent itching. Chronic tetter of the hands, scaly with thick crusts. White blisters on the face as if burnt by the sun.

Diseases—Scald head; psoriasis; scabies varicella, acne indurata, cancerous and other ulcers; herpes, eruptions following suppressed gonorrhea, sycotic eruptions, warts, moles, acne; impetigo with yellowish crusts.

Subjective—Burning pain (Ars.); sensation of heat (Bell.). Itching and heat; tingling and throbbing in ulcers, sticking sensation in the skin, gnawing sensation in the skin, Burning in miliary eruption, moist herpes with intolerable itching, that later on ulcerates. Burning, creeping, throbbing or shooting in ulcers; itching around ulcer. Herpes exedens, secreting an acrid, purulent fluid, with itching and burning; < at night.

Sticking sensation when touching the skin. Hot, painful swelling and induration of the glands.

Burning dryness of the eyes, especially on the margin of the lids. Creeping in ulcers.

Aggravation—During increase of the moon; heat of bed; washing, wet poultices.

Amelioration—Decrease of moon; all the symptoms >. Temperament—Sang-motor.

COCCULUS

Objective—Skin pale, lax, moist; adenitis; cold, hard, glandular swellings. Hard blotches containing no fluid, with a red areola around them. Wine colored spots on chest and behind the ears.

Subjective—Burning and itching, as from nettles. Itching on chest, tibia and in axillæ. Stinging pains and heat, as from needle points (Agar.), when touched, itching, < in evening when undressing (Nat. mur., Rumex. Hep., Ars., Psor.).

Aggravation—Touch, pressure, riding in a boat or carriage; undressing, itching.

Temperament—Sang-motor.

COFFEA CRUDA

Objective—Dryness of the skin in nervous diseases and coffee drinkers. Skin *excessively sensitive* (nervous individuals). Purple miliary eruption; measly spots on the skin, with dry heat at night, over-excitability and weeping. Measles, with frequent, short, dry cough (Rhus tox.). Skin over-sensitive; insomnia; dry skin; great restlessness. Scarlet rash, with weeping, lamenting, insomnia; wide awake all night, cannot close the eyes, yet very sleepy.

Subjective—Pricking, biting in the skin; forced to touch or rub the part, can't keep hands off the parts affected; especially is this true of the sexual organs. Skin very sensitive, cannot bear clothes to touch skin; better when she undresses; would like to rub or scratch affected part, but it is too sensitive.

Aggravation—Touch, rubbing; mental emotions, joy, grief; cold, open air.

Temperament—Bil-mental.

COLCHICUM

Objective—Skin dry, pale; swollen, hot, dry skin, or covered with sweat; urine scanty, dark colored. Gouty patients, with dark, thick, scanty urine. Gouty concretions. Tertiary sycosis; skin eruptions, accompanied with liver troubles. Erysipelas; smooth variety. Purple efflorescence of the face and neck and upper part of thorax; eczema in gouty patients, with a lithic condition of the blood. Eczema grows > and < as the urine improves, or as the uric acid decreases. Eczema rubrum, with scanty, beer-colored urine, or accompanied with chronic rheumatism (gouty form). The regular school palliate many cases of eczema by the use of Wine of Colchicum.

Subjective—Stinging tingling with itching.

Aggravation—Cooking food; evening, night.

Amelioration—While reposing.

These patients should drink large quantities of water.

Temperament—Bil-motor.

COLOCYNTHIS

Objective—Carbuncles, with continuous burning pain. Boils on neck and face. Corns; desquamation over whole body. Herpes of face, with crusts. Rheumatic or gouty diatheses, subject to colic; ulcers burn and itch.

Subjective—Burning, pricking, crawling, formication. Pains tearing, jerking. Carbuncles with burning pains (Carbo veg., Ars., Anth.).

Aggravation—Eating cheese; after anger and mortification.

Amelioration—Hard pressure.

Temperament—Bil-vital.

COMOCLADIA DENTATA

Objective—Red rash, resembling scarlet fever, all over the body; erysipelatous-like rash all over the body, followed by dessication and desquamation. Skin white, covered with shiny scales, or cracked and discharging a sanious fluid. Ulcers, with dry, hard edges, discharging a thick, purulent, greenish-yellow pus, having a peculiar fetid odor; parts look like raw meat, while surrounding tissue is covered with shining scales.

Subjective—Painful burning in face and arms, violent

16

itching. Tormenting itching and burning over whole body; violent itching and burning, accompanied with an erysipelatous redness.

Diseases—Malignant erysipelas; herpes; zona; leprosy, ulcers, eczema of face, scrotum, nose, with intense cor·rosive itching.

Temperament—Nervo-sanguine.

CONIUM MACULATUM

Objective—Adenitis, cancer (schirrhous), cancerous ulcers. Gangrene, bleeding ulcers (Mur. ac., Nit. ac.). Cancer of face, lips, breast; edges of ulcer tissues black, with effusion of ichor.

Hordeola of the lids. Blennorrhea of lachrymal sac. Face yellowish, pale, sallow, or bluish, bloated. Pipe cancer of the lip. Parotid and submaxillary glands swollen hard as a stone, in malignant diseases; mammary gland swollen, hard. Dull pain below left nipple; nipple contracted, dark red; glands hard, indurated about it (cancer), painful to touch; hard, painful lumps in the breast, movable for a time, but later on become fixed and bound down to the deeper tissues; tumor in mammæ with piercing pains, twinging pain; areola around nipple leaden colored. Stony hard scirrhus of the breast with piercing pains; heavy pulling in the breast; wasting and atrophy of the breast; skin flaccid, bag-like; scrofulosis, with enlargement of the lymphatics. All tumors have a stony hardness; it follows Arnica after injuries, often, or scirrhus coming on after injuries.

Herpetic eruptions forming into crusts as large as the hand; acne on the face in scrofulous subjects; eczema, humid, corroding, crusty. Old sero-purulent eruptions in old people. Petechia of old people. Blackish ulcers, with bloody, fetid discharges; ulcers, especially malignancies, bleed easily. Conium is indicated more frequently, after 50 or 60 years of age, in unmarried women, old men; scrofulous and tubercular individuals, after suppressed syphilis, or suppressed eruptions, when the lymphatics become involved; glands indurated, of a stony hardness, tendency to break down late in life. The patient is morose, easily vexed, domineering, quarrelsome, indolent.

Subjective—Burning, sticking, jerking in tumors and ulcers. Pains intolerable in affected parts. Itching, burning stitches. Single stitches in the skin. Itching, < by scratching; eczema, burning corroding, crusty.

Aggravation—Vertigo, turning in bed; scratching, at night; lying down.

It is followed well by Psorinum, Mer. iod. rub., Iod., Tub., Comocladia, Ars., Ars. iod.

Temperament—Sang-ment-nervous.

COPAIVA

Nettle rash, isolated patches, pale or bright red, with violent itching; urticaria over whole body; face red, dry, hot, with biting in the skin. Urticaria from gastric irritation, followed with fever and intolerable itching (Bell,. Aco., Puls., Bry., Nux). Post-scarlatina dropsy (Apis, Mer. sol., Ars.); case of long duration; papular or pustular skin eruptions.

Subjective—Itching, raw spots between fingers; nettle rash following a severe chill; headache, malaria; skin red, hot; delirium, drowsiness, scanty urine, with brick dust sediment. Itching, pricking in the skin. Chilblains, with intense itching. Itching in the skin with scanty urine and burning in the urethra after urinating.

Diseases—Papules and pustules in clusters; psoriasis,

urticaria; nettle rash, acne, lichen, roseola, measles, miliary eruption, scarlet rash, itch.

Temperament—Sang-lymphatic.

CORALLIUM RUB

Objective—Psoriasis; smooth, red spots on wounds, at first coral colored, changing to dark red. Flat ulcers on glans penis and inner surface (syphilitic) with yellowish, ichorous discharge. Copper-colored spots on the skin (Mer., Nit. ac., Sep., Kali iod., Ars.). Pustular eruption resembling small-pox. Flat ulcers.

Diseases—Syphilis, psoriasis, measles; profound syphilitic and psoric patients; eruptions on elbows feel like a grater.

Subjective—Profuse perspiration of genitals (Sil., Mer. viv., Psor., Thuja).

Syphilitic erosions exuding a badly smelling ichor; spasmodic whooping cough.

CORNUS (Dogwood)

Objective—Fine scarlet rash on the chest. Copious, clammy perspiration. Eczema of the genitals, with severe pruritus. Dry or moist tinea; itching of the scalp. Vesicular eruptions, with pruritus. Yellow or earthy appearance of the skin in typhoid and remittent fevers. Bilious remittents with the characteristic gastric and intestinal symptoms of this remedy.

Subjective—Heat, with violent headache; thirst, hot skin, but moist; stupor, clammy perspiration. Heat of whole surface of the skin, with itching, burning or pricking sensations. Itching in paroxysms, < at night.

Diseases—Vesicular eruptions, urticaria, miliaria, roseola, pruritus.

Aggravation—Scratching or rubbing (Coff.).

Temperament—Bil-motor.

CROCUS SATIVUS

Subjective—Scarlet redness of the whole body; scarlet spots upon the skin. Circumscribed red spots upon the face; painful suppuration of bruised parts (Amm. c., Ham., Bell. per.); old, cicatrized wounds reopen and suppurate. Lipoma and encephaloma of the scalp. Chilblains. Hæmorrhages from different parts or from the skin, black or very dark, clotted and stringy; strings hang from bleeding surfaces; acne during the menses, with dark, black or stringy, clotted flow. Face sallow in epistaxis.

Subjective—Sensation as of something alive in affected parts. Desire to be fanned, in hæmorrhages (Carbo veg.). Pricking, crawling, burning, tingling in the skin. Produces venous congestion.

Aggravation—Morning.

Amelioration—In open air, and being fanned. Pulsatilla, Sulphur, Cinchona, follows Crocus well.

CROTALUS HORRIDUS

Objective—Skin dry, stiff, like parchment; or skin hot and perspiring, yellow color of the whole body. Acute jaundice from rheumatic causes. Petechia like blotches or purple spots; yellow, green or bluish spots. Purpura hæmorrhagica. Blisters with livid spots over the body; erythematous spots, which soon vesicate, then form pustules, dessicate and desquamate. Scarlet erythema of the whole body. Erysipelas of the face; herpes on the scrotum; eruption about the mouth and eyes, herpetic in form. Burns and scalds, threatening erysipelas and gangrene, sloughing ulcers. Pustular eruptions, after vaccination. Old scars break open (Caust.). Hot swellings with cold skin, and a sickly appearance. Dissecting wounds. followed by malignant erysipelas. Chilblains with gangrene (Carbo veg.) Morbilli, malignant, purpuric form; scarlatina, with great intoxication of the whole system. Vomiting and general collapse, coma or convulsions; throat livid; rapid swelling, great edema; head thrown back, eruption patchy, livid, petechial; pulse quick, feeble, epistaxis; face dusky; tenacious mucus from the mouth and nostrils; breathing irregular and jerky. Secondary infection. Low typhoid states. Hæmorrhages from internal organs.

Subjective—Itching stinging all over; urticaria.

Diseases—Syphilis, ulcers becoming gangrenous. Pemphigus with a low typhoid condition present. Dropsy, cardiac, hepatic and renal; anthrax, gangrene, erysipelas phlegmonous. Dissecting wounds, with erysipelas following. Pustulous eruptions after vaccination. Burns and scalds, hepatic jaundice, malignant pustules; herpes on the scrotum; morbilla, scarlatina maligna, apoplexy, convulsions in inebriates; hæmorrhagic diathesis; blood flows from every orifice in the body. Compare with Lach., Bryonia, Ars., Naja, Elaps cor., Carbo veg.

Temperament—Nervo-bilious.

CROTON TIGLIUM

Objective—Erysipelas, with excessive itching. Scarlet redness of the skin, with vesicles. Red, moist spots exuding moisture about the scrotum, or on left thigh. Eczema over the whole body, even to soles of the feet. Eczema of the face and genitals, more frequently in children. Vesicular eruption, with burning, itching, stinging and redness of the skin; sero-purulent exudation; vesicopustular eruption similar to Rhus tox. Intense erythema with vesicles and pustules.

Subjective—Itching of the scrotum very intense, followed by a voluptuous sensation, < scratching, > gentle rubbing (Coff.). *Itching followed by painful burning.* Itching with painful burning and redness of the skin. Vesicular eruption on an erythematous base with itching, burning and stinging (Rhus tox.). Sensation as if hidebound.

Diseases—Erysipelatous eruption; erythema. Pustular eruptions, impetigo. Prurigo, eczema, herpes (Rhus poisoning as an antidote); glandular affections.

Aggravation—Scratching, from sweets and from fruits.
Amelioration—Gentle rubbing.

CUNDURANGO

Objective—Pustular eruptions between eyebrows, side of nose, tip of tongue, right cheek, abdomen. Open epithelioma, erythematous blotches on face and body, eczema; rhagades usually present. oozing out a fetid fluid; syphilitic dyscrasia. Indolent ulcers, with hard, callous edges, discharge fetid, sanious. Old ulcers become cancerous. Old, obstinate, foul, ichorous ulcers. Varicose syphilitic ulcers; also, ulcers of small-pox. Open carcinoma; open epithelioma, with stinging, burning.

Diseases—Epithelioma, erysipelas, eczema. Rhagades discharging ichorous fluid, irritating the surrounding parts. Scrofulosis, small-pox, syphilis, teleangeiectasis, open ulcers, lupus-vulgaris, fissures in muco-cutaneous outlets (Anac. oc.); sore cracks in corners of the mouth.

CUPRUM ACETICUM

Objective—Leprous eruptions, without itching. Spasmodic symptoms, cramps in the legs (Sulph.). Contractions of fingers and toes. Spasmodic disease, whooping cough, etc. Acute exanthemata when checked in the stage of eruption. Pulse, quick, small, irregular. Skin over whole body cyanotic, convulsions and severe spasmodic symptoms follow. In suppressed scarlet fever or measles with brain symptoms following, threatening paralysis of brain.

Temperament—Sang-ment-motor.

CYCLAMEN EUROPÆUM

Objective—Eczema of the face; bright red spots on thighs. Facial eruptions of children. Best indicated in leuco-phlegmatic individuals who are anæmic, easily fatigued, pale, chlorotic, peevish, irritable, morose. Eruptions painless. Patient never thirsty (Puls., Apis).

Subjective—Itching leaves a numb sensation. Itching, pricking, < night in bed, > scratching, but it leaves a numb sensation, or itching disappears to reappear at another place; gnawing, stinging, itching, eruptions following suppressed menses with headache, palpitation and vertigo.

Aggravation—Afternoon, evening (Puls.); eating fat foods (Puls).

Amelioration—Moving, walking.

Temperament—Sang-motive.

DIGITALIS

Objective—Cyanotic condition of the whole body in heart affections or from bad heart action. Face pale, deathlike appearance, or bluish red. Blueness of the face, eyelids, lips, tongue; veins distended; surface of the body cold, pulse slow, intermittent (every fourth beat). Black comedones on the face; pores of the skin dark, even black; pimples on the back, rash on the hands, desquamation, anasarca of the extremities, white, elastic swelling of the whole body, or of dropsical parts. Much flabbiness and edema. Gouty nodosities.

Subjective—Corrosive itching, darting; gnawing itching increasing to an intolerable burning. Creeping all over the skin. Skin painful to touch. Titillation in affected parts.

Aggravation—Warm room (Puls., China, Carbo veg.); sitting erect; motion.

Temperament—Nervo-lymphatic.

DOLICHOS PRURIENS

Objective—Dry, tettery eruptions on anus and legs resembling zona. Prurigo in jaundice, skin yellow in spots, or all over, with itching excessive at night.

Subjective—Itching without any eruptions. Violent itching all over the body, with invisible eruption; scratching increases eruption. Terrible itching over the whole body, with swelling of the face and lips, yet compelled to scratch constantly without relief; ten days later the skin desquamates in small, fine scales; as soon as desquamation takes place itching and swelling returns. Herpes zoster in rings.

Aggravation—Scratching; night, in bed; during pregnancy.

DROSERA

Objective—Acts on pneumogastric and respiratory tract; eruption like measles; black pores on the chest, shoulders and chin. Eruptions with painful soreness and stinging. Ulcers with burning and bleeding; cutting pains; pus bloody, thin, watery, ichorous, < later part of night and morning. Usually with spasmodic whistling, laryngeal cough, < after midnight.

Subjective—Burning after rubbing. Itching, pricking, burning, gnawing, stinging, scratching, < undressing, or from cold.

Aggravation—Undressing, getting warm in bed, after midnight. (Complementary to Nux vom.).

Amelioration—Walking, rubbing.

DULCAMARA

Objective—Pale face, with circumscribed red cheeks (Cham., Phos., Sang.). Humid eruptions on the cheeks. Pimples and little ulcers around the mouth, with tearing pain when moving the part. Thick, brown, yellowish crusts on the face, forehead, temples and chin. Thick, brown, herpetic crusts on the face, with reddish borders, bleeding when scratched. White blotches with red areola on the arms and thighs. Suppressed eruptions. Herpes, oozing after scratching. Rash before the menses, with much sexual excitement. Herpes of the vulva during menses, or worse every cold change of weather. Glands of the neck swollen, sensitive. Exostosis on upper part of right tibia, with bluish red spots. Suppurating nodes. Skin hot and dry in fevers, or skin sensitive to cold; have urticaria or some other eruption when they take cold. Vesicular eruption as large as a pea, containing a yellow fluid and on a red inflamed base (Rhus, Canth.), covering the whole body except the face. Pemphigus. Tetter oozing a watery fluid; bleeds when scratching. Itching pustules, which cease to itch when crusted over; sensitive to touch; < washing. Nettle rash over whole body without fever. Eczema scrofulosum over the whole body; glandular enlargements; exuding vesicles on the face and extremities. Thick, brown herpes with a red border; glands swollen; yellow, suppurating herpes; scaly, round herpes. Herpetic eruption associated with fetid perspiration. Suppressed itch. Herpes, preputialis, easily bleeding; brown, dry or humid, or furfuraceous, red, pale red, or with a red areola; callous or warty growths on the skin. Warts, fleshy or large and smooth on hands and face; large, flat warts. Painless ulcers, hard, sometimes sensitive, < night, from wet or cold (Rhus tox.).

Subjective—Burning when rubbed. Burning itching, like the rapid crawling of insects. Sticking itching in various parts of the body. Sensitive to cold, moisture. Burning in the genitals. Pains coming on from cold or wet (Rhus tox.).

Aggravation—Lying on back (Mer. sol.); stooping (Rhus); cold, *wet weather*, sweat, suppressed eruptions, suppressed menstruation.

Amelioration—Lying on side, moving (Rhus, Ferr. met., Puls.). Complementary to Baryta carb.

Temperament—Bil-motive.

EUPHORBIUM

Objective—Boils, chronic erysipelatous eruptions. Pea sized yellow vesicles on the face, with swelling of the part. Scarlet red streaks on the forearm; old, indolent ulcers; red inflammatory swelling of the cheeks, with sensation of burning heat. Eruption on hairy and covered parts (Thuja). Erysipelas with bullæ. Straw-colored pustules on the hands, face, chin. Impetigo, with burning itching.

Subjective—Sensation as of a thin cord under the skin. Biting, stinging, gnawing, burning, itching; burning itching induces scratching. Biting exanthema. Torpid ulcers with lancinating pains; gangrenous ulcers biting in ulcers, < in morning, on getting near the stove; < motion, touch.

Aggravation—Contact.

EUPHRASIA

Objective—Fine eruption around the nose and eyes; eyes sensitive to light; eyes weep easily from the effects of light or dust. Streaming hot, burning tears from the eyes (Rhus tox.). Measles with the catarrhal symptoms of this remedy (eye and nose symptoms). Coryza, frontal headache, cough, catarrhal symptoms.

Subjective—Burning, formication and numbness of the part. Shooting stitches here and there in the skin all during the night. Bad effects of contusions (Am. carb.).

Aggravation—Evening, when touched (Hep.).

Temperament—Sang-mental.

ELATERIUM

Objective—Whole surface of an orange yellow color, white of eyes yellowish tinge. Urine stains diaper an orange color. Stools yellow (icterus neonatorum). Burning and itching over the affected parts. Measles, followed by dysentery. Post-scarlatina dropsy. Urticaria with intolerable itching.

Subjective—Intolerable itching in icterus; > rubbing.

Amelioration—Rubbing, urticaria.

FERRUM METALLICUM

Objective—Skin, pale, sallow, yellow, dirty, withered, flabby; even mucous membranes are pale and bloodless. Red parts become white, lips, tongue, membranes of the mouth. Patient often so anæmic suffers from a severe vertigo. Hæmorrhagic diathesis. Yellowish brown spots on the skin, sore to touch. Dirty, brown discoloration of the skin (Sep., Iod.). Inflammation and suppuration of dark hepatic spots. Scarlatina, sometimes indicated in the desquamative stage; anasarca. Ulcers pale, edematous.

(It is complementary to Alum and China.) Pale, bloated appearance of the skin after hæmorrhages. Each day the skin seems to become paler.

Subjective—Burning sensation, with pain as if excoriated when touched.

Aggravation—At night, at rest.

Amelioration—Walking slowly about; summer.

Temperament—Sang-mental.

FLUORIC ACID

Objective—Skin sallow or grayish white. Elevated red blotches, varicose veins and ulcers, obstinate, long standing cases, in women who have borne children. Flat nævus in children about the temples; capillary aneurism. Skin tubercles about forehead and face; elevated red blotches on the palms of the hands; squamous eruptions on the body (psoriasis guttata). Syphilitic erosions and exostosis, with nightly pains, boils, carbuncles, pustules. Dry, cutaneous eruptions. Old cicatrices become red around the edges, covered or surrounded by itching vesicles. Bed sores. Indicated in old people with sallow skin, who are emaciating constantly; diseases of the long bones. Psoro-syphilitic patients. Complementary to Silicea.

Subjective—Excessive sweat upon the feet (Sil., Baryta c.); ulcers > by washing or bathing them with cold water. Soreness between the toes (Sil.). Soreness in all corns. Onychia, with itching pains (Hep.). Burning pain in a small spot in the skin. Sensation as if a burning vapor was emitted from the pores of the skin. Ulcers painful, < warmth, > cold water. Itching of cicatrices of ulcers.

Aggravation—Warmth, ulcers; night; bone diseases.

Amelioration—Daytime, cold water.

Temperament—Bil-motor.

16

GAMBOGIA

Subjective—Violent itching on various parts of the skin, accompanied with a pleasant sensation, > by gentle friction. After scratching burning and ulcerative pain. Biting like ants over the whole body, < evening and nights. Itching blisters on hands, first pale, then red.

GELSEMIUM

Objective—Indicated in children, young people and women. Skin hot, dry in fevers. Papular eruptions, like measles, on the face. Measles, with catarrhal symptoms predominant (Euph.); spasmodic sneezing, dry, tickling cough (Rhus). Erysipelas of a mild variety; erythema and papules. Measles, with torpor, drowsiness and high fevers, jerking of the muscles, and loss of muscular power. Scarlet fever, with stupor and flushed face (Bell.). Asthenic forms of scarlet fever; fever intense with nervous erethism during the prodromal stage, followed by great prostration of muscular power, brain symptoms grave; pulse frequent, soft, weak; heat, with languor, drowsiness, face flushed, heavy looking (Bapt.); eyes suffused, delirium of low form. Eruption apt to recede.

Subjective—Itching preventing sleep; after scratching, raw and sore, followed by blisters.

Aggravation—Mental emotion, bad news; damp weather, when thinking about his ailments.

Temperament—Nervo-bilious.

GRAPHITES

Objective—Graphites is an anti-psoric, sycotic and anti-syphilitic remedy. It is also typically a tubercular remedy; most of the skin symptoms, however, are of a latent, syphilitic or tubercular character. It is suitable in infant life and old age. Skin harsh, dry, thickened, rough, fissured, disposed to chafing. Skin inclined to crack (Tub., Pet., Hep., Nat.-mur., Kali sulph., Kali iod.). Fissures deep, bleeding or oozing out a sticky fluid (shallow, Tub., Nat. mur.). (Moist Pet., Graph.). Raw moist places between the fingers and on the face. Every injury suppurates (Hep.). Cracks or fissures on fingers, hands, toes, lips, behind the ears, anus, labia, nipples, especially in nursing women, with or without any discharge, sometimes only bleeding slightly. Erysipelas, beginning in face and spreading in all directions; it follows Rhus sometimes. Erysipelas assuming a vesicular appearance, like Rhus tox., and exudes a transparent honey-like secretion, or assumes a chronic form. Eczema of hands, fissure form. Eczema behind the ears, moist, oozes a watery, transparent, sticky fluid. Eczema behind the ears, raw, bleeding easily, pus thick, creamy, smelling like tubercular pus or old cheese (Hep.). Moist, offensive, semi-purulent with fissures (Pet.). Dry fissured, bleeding, but fissures not deep (Tub.). Eczema with profuse serous exudations of a sticky consistency, in fleshy blondes. Small, red, itching pimples tipped with pus. Intertrigo with profuse serous discharge. Erythema dark, bluish, fissured, bleeding, bathed with a sticky, viscid secretion, or skin dry, harsh, rough, with intense itching; after digging into it with the nails, weeps profusely the sticky, honey-like discharge. Eczema on the genitals, face, scalp, behind the ears, hands, fingers, toes, calves of the legs, bends of the knees, flexures of the body. Skin thick as leather, dry, rough, harsh, cracks open when flexing the part; < snowy weather or wet weather. Graphites eruptions usually disappear during the summer or hot weather, and appear the first cold weather in the fall, especially the first snowy weather. Eczema of laborers, tanners, workers in water, plasterers, masons, painters, weavers, dry goods clerks, washerwomen, dyers, etc. Scald head with glutinous discharge, forming crusts; even the crusts crack and ooze a viscid secretion. Felons, boils, onychia, or paronychia, hang nails or nails brittle, hard, horny, break and split easily (Sil., Tub., Sulph.). Herpes exuding a sticky matter. Leprous spots, coppery, annular, raised; on face, ears, legs, feet, toes, nose, nostrils. Crusty, scaly ulcers, with fetid pus; tubercles, or tubercular ulcers; callous spots on feet, toes, hands.

Diseases—Herpes, boils, erysipelas, erythema, callosities, zona, eczema, fissures, intertrigo, ulcers, dandruff, felons, lichen, prurigo, leprosy.

Subjective—Severe itching, < night, cold or wet weather. Violent itching and burning, itching relieved by hard scratching, followed by oozing; when crusts form and become dry, itching returns. Prurigo in children, with raw places on the skin (intertrigo); corrosive itching. Burning, throbbing after scratching, or tearing, burning, smarting, stinging, itching; the only relief from the itching is by tearing the flesh or hard rubbing. The patient rubs the part with a piece of board or some hard substance until it bleeds or weeps the peculiar sticky discharge.

Aggravation—Night; snowy weather; after and during menstruation; when constipated. Water applied to skin, wet weather.

Amelioration—Dry, high altitude; hot, summer weather.

Constipation a constant symptom; > to be given before Sulph., than after. Is followed well by Lyc., Puls., Sep., Tub. It cannot be compared with any special remedy, as it stands out alone. If any comparison is to be made, it will be frequently Tuberculinum.

Temperament— Sang-lymphatic.

GRINDELIA ROBUSTA

Objective—Epidemic rash, like roseola, suffusing face, neck, and often the whole body, with severe burning and itching (Rhus tox. poisoning). Bites of insects, flea bites (Led.). Purplish blue ulcer over the tibia, very long and deep.

Subjective—Pruritus affecting vulva and vagina, from leucorrhea, aphthæ.

HAMAMELIS VIRGINICA

Objective—Adapted to venous congestions hæmorrhages from every orifice of the body; nose, lungs, bowels, uterus, rectum. Venous congestion, varicose ulcers, varicose veins. Bruised, sore feeling in affected parts (Am. carb.). Hæmorrhage, passive (Crot. tig.). profuse, dark, painless. Varicose veins of the lower extremities during pregnancy, with crampy pains at night, preventing sleep (Sulph.). Hæmorrhagic purpura. Ulcers with stinging, pricking pains. Varicose ulcers, flat, deep, very dark; skin surrounding the ulcer blue or black, oozing dark blood, burning, stinging or biting in the ulcer. Chilblains always bluish. Boils, abscesses, resulting from falls. Great ecchymosis after injury, color blue or black (Arnica greenish blue). Petechia and ecchymosis in small-pox, typhoid, scarlatina. Passive congestion and venous stagnation in skin and mucous membranes. Complementary to Ferr.

Aggravation—Touch, motion.

Temperament—Bil-motive.

HEKLA LAVA

Objective—Exostosis of the tibia; nodosities very large with severe, continuous pain. Necrosis of the whole bone. This remedy has cured many cases of necrosis of

17

the bone when an operation seemed unavoidable. Caries of the bones of the feet. Osteo-sarcoma, exostosis, periostitis, rachitis. No good proving of this remedy has yet been made. Symptoms clinical, principally.

HEPAR SULPH

Objective—Torpid, lymphatic constitutions, light hair, fair complexion, slow to act. Muscles soft, flabby. Diseases induced by Mercury. It hastens or aborts suppuration. Ulcers or herpes surrounded by little papules or pustules; the slightest injury suppurates (Graph.). Boils *very sensitive*, discharging much yellow pus. Eczema on the face and genitals, discharging much pus. Intertrigo with surface bathed with pus; pus in excess always an abundance; parts tender, sensitive; pus smells like old cheese; very sensitive to cold and to touch. Pustules large, yellow, pouring out abundant yellow pus, bad smelling like rotten eggs. Ulcers bleed easily when slightly touched, smell sour, putrid, like old cheese. Eczema spreading by new pimples on its outer border. Erythema in the folds of the muscles, groins, bends of the body. Nettle rash, sensitive to cold. Urticaria in children and young people, more frequently indicated in this disease than any other remedy; < touch, cold, draft of air, undressing, rubbing or scratching; light blondes, patients of a latent, syphilitic or tubercular diathesis, who take cold easily, and as soon as skin becomes chilled urticaria appears. (Ulcers sensitive to touch, bleed easily, have splintery pains (Nit. ac.), accompanied with burning or stinging and soreness. Margins elevated, spongy, with granulations in the centre; crusts soft, friable, easily broken, much pus under them, bleeding easily, yellowish in color, greasy, easily broken up or torn off, when they bleed easily.

Children cross, irritable. Lymphatic glands usually enlarged, with a tendency to form abscesses; discharge copious, yellow or creamy colored, thick, bad smelling, bland; lesion sensitive to touch, and bleeds easily.

Subjective—Burning, itching in bends of the extremities; biting and pulsating in abscesses and boils; sensation as if ulcerating in the skin. Violent itching in the bends of elbows and different parts of body. Over-sensitiveness to pain (Coff.). Pains ulcerative, splinter-like (Nit. ac.).

The least cold produces laryngeal hoarseness, or hoarseness and rawness in the throat, with a scratching, scraping feeling. Children who are subject to cough on the least exposure to cold. Nettle rash, with violent itching and stinging, that disappears as the body becomes warm. Felon, or suppuration about the fingers and finger nails with throbbing pain, hot burning; throbbing pain, sensitive to touch, < by cold applications, > by heat.

Aggravation—Mercury, cold, touch, lying on painful side.

Amelioration—Warmth in general; damp, wet weather; also, better covering up warm (Sil.). Complementary to Calendula in injuries.

Temperament—Sanguine-lymphatic.

HIPPOZAENIN (Glandium)

Objective—Putrid bed sores. Erythema, erysipelas or phlegmonous processes. Abscesses, pustules and ulcers spread extensively over the surface.

Malignant erysipelas, with profuse flow of pus, or attended with the formation of much pus and destruction of the part. Red spots on the skin soon change into pustules, similar to small-pox. Pemphigus, with blebs soon filling with pus (Hep.), but Hepar is bland and non-malignant, while this of Hippozaenin is corrosive and malignant in its nature. Pustules the size of peas arise in large numbers which soon burst, discharging a thick muco pus of an offensive odor. Large abscesses, with glands about them, enlarged and swollen; obstinate syphilitic, sores; ulcers show no disposition to heal, and of a dirty white color. Sinuous and fistulous ulcers, secreting an offensive, watery pus. Pustules containing caseous, purulent contents (Hep.). Malignant phagedenic skin diseases.

Lupus exedens. Fluctuating tumors in muscular tissues. Malignant diphtheria, with a black, sooty colored membrane.

Subjective—Probably no nosode brings with it such death dealing, or has such destructive properties as this one. The tongue dry, covered with a black, sooty coating, unable to speak.

Diseases—Malignant pustules, diphtheria, bed sores, small-pox, plague, elephantiasis, syphilitic ulcers, scarlet fever, measles, carbuncle, boils, abscesses, erysipelas phlegmonous, lupus exedens, fluctuating tumors, icterus, murrain in cattle.

HYDRASTIS

Objective—Skin jaundiced, greenish yellow color. Yellowish looking vesicles filled with a limpid fluid. Hyperidrosis, offensive, especially of the axillæ and genitals. Obstinate cases of intertrigo in children. Fissures around mucous outlets. Ulcers with indolent granulations; unhealthy, scanty pus; scrofulous or cachectic individuals.

Subjective—Small-pox, itching, tingling of skin, great redness, swelling and aching of the skin, very sore throat, intense aching in the back and legs; pustules dark, great prostration. Face covered with a fine rash in confluent small-pox. Chronic ulcers arising from contusions, lacerated wounds, burns, scalds; pricking pain in ulcers on moving the part. In small-pox, when it is indicated, it is said to quiet the irritation of the skin at once, remove the odor, prevents pitting, to a very great degree, and destroys the contagious character of the disease; discharges stringy, ropy (Kali b.).

Aggravation—Slightest touch causes ulcers to bleed (Mer. cor., Hep., Nit. ac., Ham.).

HYPERICUM

Objective—Eruption like nettle rash, < at 4 P. M. (Lyc.). Punctured wounds, from nails, splinters, needles, or sharp-pointed instruments; pressure on nerve endings or nerve trunks after injuries or surgical operations. Shock from injuries or surgical operations (Staph., Arn.). Injury to fingers and toes; often prevents tetanus. Hard, dry, yellow crusts form on wounds, or open sores.

Subjective—Tetanus after injuries. Spasms and convulsions after injuries. Epileptic convulsions after wounds. Violent smarting in the skin, bad effects of spinal injuries or concussions.

It may follow Arnica in injuries.

Aggravation—At 4 P. M.

Temperament—Nervous.

IGNATIA

Objective—Ulcers, painless; discharge scanty, burning, < from slightest touch, > hard pressure.

Subjective—Oversensitive to pain (Coff., Hep.). Tingling as of ants in the skin. Great sensitiveness to drafts of air. Twitching and jerking in the muscles and skin when lying quiet. Burning in ulcers. Itching relieved by rubbing or scratching, biting, pricking in the nerve endings in the skin, as if bitten by an insect; nervous reflexes cause most of the skin irritation. Adapted to highly nervous, sensitive, hysterical women. Fine pricking like flea bites (Inula).

Aggravation—Mental emotions, grief, joy, cold drafts, coffee, tobacco.

Amelioration—By gentle pressure, rubbing the part gently; warmth, walking.

Temperament—Nervo-bilious.

IODINE

Objective—Scrofulous subjects with dark hair and eyes (Nit. ac.).

Skin rough, dry, dirty yellow or clammy, moist, cool. Eruptions furfuraceous, humid. Tertiary syphilis with ulcerations of the skin. Eruption like scarlet rash; glandular indurations; skin dry, rough, thickened, like parchment. Eruptions brownish or yellowish brown in color. Greasy scales, dropsical swellings; indurations of the glands; glands hypertrophied, hard as a stone (Con.).

Goitre, hard to touch, firm, unyielding. Ulcers bleeding profusely, destitute of feeling, or hard, spongy and sensitive; discharge copious, bloody, corroding, thin, watery. Abscesses profuse, suppurative, pus copious (Hep.).

Subjective—Violent itching, nettle rash, about the knees. Burning itching, drawing burning. Emaciation general in most diseases.

Aggravation—Warmth; wrapping up the head (Sil.); (reverse, Hep., Psor.).

Amelioration—Cold; uncovering; rubbing.

Temperament—Bil-motor.

IPECACUANHA

Objective—Nausea, the keynote to this remedy; does not entirely disappear in skin diseases. The hæmorrhages are bright red and passive; they may be from any orifice of the body. Miliary eruptions; miliaria rubra, with nausea or colic and dyspnea; miliary rash on forehead, temples, cheeks. Eruption suppressed or tardy in making its appearance with vomiting and oppression of the chest. Erysipelas, the eruption suddenly disappears with vomiting. Vascular erethism with tardy development of the eruption in exanthematous diseases, with constriction of the chest, dyspnea, or vomiting and diarrhœa.

Subjective—Pricking, burning itching.

Aggravation—Motion; winter, dry weather.

Temperament—Sang-lymphatic.

IRIS VERSICOLOR

Objective—Tinea capitis; crusta lactea; prurigo; eczema of the face. Pustular eruptions on the nose, cheeks, face, secreting a bloody pus. Obstinate lepra vulgaris on the arms. Herpes zoster on the right side of the body. Psoriasis; irregular patches on knees, elbows and body, with shining scales. Will sometimes abort felons.

Temperament—Bilious.

VIOLA TRICOLOR

Objective—Scurfs on the head with unbearable burning, < at night. Tinea capitis, with frequent involuntary urination. Impetigo of face and hairy scalp; thick incrustations, pouring out copious, thick, yellow pus, which agglutinates the hair. Seborrheic eczema; eczema of the scalp. Crusts dry, light cream or lemon color, with no discharge; hair falls out. Milk crust, with burning itching, < at night; pus viscid, yellow. Eruption soon becomes pustular, which sooner or later forms yellowish brown crusts; much itching at all stages. Skin eruptions of scrofulous children; impetigo contagiosa with yellow-ish.,crusts; urine smells like cat's urine. Ichorous ulcers with severe itching.

Subjective—Cutting, stinging in the skin. Tingling in the skin; unbearable burning in the scurfs on the head; milk crust with burning and itching.

Aggravation—Worse lying on the painful side (Bry.); open air.

JUGLANS CINEREA

Objective—Erythema nodosum; large spots, varying in size from that of a dollar to a man's hand. Erysipelas of the extremities as well as on the body. Eruptions upon the body, face and anus; painful itching, causing an irresistible desire to tear off the crusts. Confluent pustules, thickly set; while drying up on one part of the body they were breaking out fresh in another. Impetigo upon the chin, which had been torn and broken, producing hard crusts, which nearly covered the entire surface. Pustular eruptions. Lichen, lividus; eczema, chronic of the hands, disappearing in one place and appearing in another, discharge ichorous and semi-purulent, causing intolerable itching and soreness. Eczema confluent, pustular forms; changing into thick crusts with unbearable pain and tension about them. Herpes circinatus about the chin, very large patches.

Subjective—Tension and pain in the lesions, especially in the thick crusts of this remedy. Itching painful, intolerable in eczema.

Diseases—Eczema, ecthyma, erysipelas, herpes circinatus, impetigo, pemphigus eruptions, brownish or yellowish brown (Sep., Iod.).

KALI BICHROMICUM

Objective—Eruptions on face like small-pox; pustules

like small-pox; pustules about the roots of the nails, spreading to the wrists. Skin hot, dry, red in inflammations; bright red, shiny eruption all over the body. Measles, hoarse, distressing; croupy cough on the appearance of the eruption.

Papular eruption began as a spot in the calf of the leg and spread all over the body; large papular elevation, irregular, like measles, but more raised, with intense and excessive burning and itching like fire (Ars., Rhus, Canth.), especially at night. Herpes after taking cold, with fluent coryza and bronchial symptoms peculiar to this remedy. Pustular syphiloderma. Impetigo pustules. Ulcers deep yellow, dry, oval, edges overhanging, bright red areola, base hard, ulcer becoming deeper, blackish points in the centre; cicatrix depressed. Ulcers of syphilitic origin, deep, with hard edges on genitals, throat, uvula, nose, septum, etc.; discharge stringy, ropy, yellowish green. Head and scalp covered with dry, red, scaly patches at root of hair (Nat. mur.). Ulcers of the tongue, or any mucous membrane, yellowish in color; discharge stringy, thread like, watery, corroding discharges. Light haired persons; fat, chubby, short-necked children, disposed to croupy cough; deep ulcers in the fauces, pains at root of nose, discharge of clinkers or ropy mucus or pus from the nose.

Subjective—Itching and heat at night, followed by a papular eruption, nightly bone pains (Mer., Kali iod., Nit. ac.). Burning and stinging in the skin; heat and itching in the skin, < at night, < heat, > cold (Mer.).

Diseases—Diphtheritic formations in nose and throat. Ulcers, syphilitic or non-syphilitic; papules, pustules, vesicles, boils, impetigo, zona, lupus, chronic forms; diseases of the bones, acne.

Aggravation—Heat; night, summer or hot weather.

Amelioration—Skin symptoms, > cold (reverse, Ars., Pet., Alum, Cal. c., Hep., Psor.).
Temperament—Sang-vital.

KALI BROMATUM

Objective—Adapted to large, fleshy people, to children especially. Skin cold, blue spotted in severe acute diseases. Moist eczema of the legs, with pityriasis of the scalp. Slightly elevated, smooth, red patches, like urticaria, but with hardened bases; in lymphatic constitutions, acne simplex and indurata; large, red, angry looking papules or papules becoming pustular; bluish, red papules or pustules on face, neck, not very sore or sensitive, leaving scars and pitting on healing. Small boils, tubercles; large, indolent, painful pustules (Carbo veg.).

Subjective—Voluptuous itching, tingling and irritation in external genital organs. Pruritus of the genitals, from reflex uterine and ovarian irritation. Nervous restlessness and twitchings; can't sit still. Parts feel as if growing large. Burning in the vulva; heat in the genitals.
Temperament—Sang-vital.

KALI CARBONICUM

Objective—Adapted to dark haired, lax fibre, fleshy people; tubercular diathesis. Chronic dryness of the skin; deficient perspiration (Sulph.). Tubercular acne (Nat. mur., Phos., Tub., Sulph., Psor., Hep.). Tubercles small, natural color of the skin, do not undergo much change. Eczema usually dry, but when scratched exudes moisture.

Subjective—Burning, itching herpes, < scratching. Bleeding, burning, boring ulcers; ichorous thin, corroding discharge, watery or bloody. Varices with tingling, pricking pains in hæmorrhoids, darting stitches in the skin. Tubercular patients who are always tired and who suffer constantly with backache.

Aggravation— < before menses; from cold.

Amelioration— < resting, pressure, company.

Temperament—Bil-vital.

KALMIA

Objective—Adapted to sycotic, rheumatic or gouty people; gouty concretions in the joints; red and inflamed spots on the skin; erysipelas similar to Rhus tox., with oppressed breathing. Angry looking red spots on the skin. Cracked lips, with dry skin. Eruptions with accompanying rheumatic and gouty symptoms.

Subjective—Stabbing, stitching pains in the skin, shifting and changing position, running downward; sensation of rigidity in the skin.

KALI IODATUM

Objective—Scrofulous or syphilitic patients; emaciation and loss of appetite (Iod). Purpura hæmorrhagica; discharge from mucous surfaces thin, ichorous, corrosive, greenish. Osteo-nodes, periosteal pains and inflammation, caries and necrosis. Syphilitic nodes and synovitis, glands swollen or suppurate; discharge thin, corrosive or curdy. Atrophy of the glands, mammæ, testicles, etc. Ulcers vegetate, bleed easily, deep, involving all the tissues, even the bones. Rupia syphilitica. Condylomata, long standing, or following suppressed chancre. Bubo hard, with curdy, offensive discharge. Ulceration of nose, mouth, throat, with corroding, burning discharge. Bone swellings and enlargements, nightly bone or periosteal pains. Tubercular pustules on the face; roseola on the chest, tertiary syphilis, roseola spots, erythema nodosum; herpes the size of a dime on the cheeks; pityriasis capitals; boils large, hard, red, suppurating, leaving scars, appearing on the neck, face, shoulders, chest, back, scalp. Pustulous eruptions umbilicated and leaving scars. Erythematous eruptions of a syphilitic origin; ecthyma, thick, dark green, plates or crusts, oozing yellowish, greenish, ichorous pus. Ulcers dark red, well defined edges, copious discharges, < by cold, > by heat (reverse, Mer.). Ulcers often yellowish colored (Kali bich.); deep, cavernous, filled with much broken down material, offensive and ichorous pus, frequently without pain, tenderness or soreness, and accompanied with general emaciation and loss of appetite. Syphilitic, neoplasm or gummæ tumors in the muscular tissues; round, movable at first, but later on become fixed and break into a sluffing ulcer, destroying all the tissues lying beneath, even to the bones. Undermining ulcers. Tubercular syphilitic skin eruptions, with a tendency to break down into an ulcer, with all the characteristics of this remedy.

Subjective—Gnawing in the bones and periosteum < at night; gnawing, boring, tearing pains, > external warmth. Emaciation, with night sweats. Painful syphilitic nodes.

Aggravation—Night; cold.

Temperament—Sang-vital.

KALI MURIATICUM

Objective—Intertrigo of infants; chapped hands or lips from cold (Tub., Graph., Pet.). Blisters arising from burns, filled with a light colored lymph. Vesicles, with sero-fibrous contents; herpes zoster. Eczema, arising from vaccination, with greenish or brownish-yellow crusts. Barber's itch. Measles, with hoarse cough, glandular swellings, furred tongue, white or greenish coating; diarrhœa, with light-colored stools. Variola.

Abscess, carbuncles, boils in the second stage, when

interstitial exudation takes place. Causes swelling to disappear before pus forms. Obstinate eczema of the head and face of children. Ingrown toe nails, warts on the hands.

KALI SULPH

Objective—Very similar to Pulsatilla in its action on the skin. Abundant scaling of the epidermis. Promotes desquamation after erysipelas. Accelerates removal of scabs in small-pox. Epithelial cancer, with thin, yellow, serous discharge. Eczema, with yellow, sticky, watery discharge. Nails very imperfect, showing arrested or slow growth.

Subjective—Burning itching in papular eruption, exuding pus-like moisture. Desquamation of fine scales, with itching and stinging intensely; > first by bathing in cold water, then by heat. Itching pimples, rising singly on the skin.

Temperament—Sang-phlegmatic.

KREOSOTUM

Objective—Eczema, dry as well as moist, on any part of the body; large, greasy, pock-marked pustules all over the body; skin tense, shining, deep red; greasy moisture. Watery or sero-purulent herpes on the backs of the hands and finger joints, ears, elbows; < evenings and open air. Old ulcers, painful, putrid. Red, scaly skin in the bends of the knees, like herpes.

Subjective—Itching, with violent burning after scratching, on the extremities, while on the abdomen it is relieved by scratching. Small wounds bleed profusely. Corrosive itching in the vulva, due to discharges or secretions from uterus and vagina; burning and swelling of the labia; violent itching between labia and thighs. All discharges, even hæmorrhages, corrosive and irritating. Sick, suffering expression of the face in children; eyes sunken, with blue rings about them; fretful, morose, peevish, ill-tempered; screams much at night during dentition; caries of the teeth as soon as they come through. Temperament—Bil-motor.

LAC CANINUM

Objective—Mental symptoms marked; fear of dogs, absent-minded, forgetful, despondent; thinks disease incurable; imagines she is unclean or filthy, etc. Countenance pale and careworn. Chancre on the glans penis, with fungoid growth or cauliflower excrescence. Shining, glazed appearance of ulcer on skin, and wrist; [syphilis]. Bright red, scarlet eruption on face and chest in diphtheria; grayish or yellowish-colored ulcers, foul smelling, diphtheritic in their nature. Herpetic eruption in the axillæ, with light brownish scabs, painful when walking. Red, glistening appearance in ulcerations. Small-pox, with diphtheritic symptoms.

Temperament—Bil-motor.

LACHESIS

Objective—Dark, gangrenous vesicles, bullæ or blebs. Malignant, dark blue or black pustules extremely sensitive to touch. Carbuncles of a bluish or purplish appearance. Can't even tolerate a bandage or slightest touch. Simple or phlegmonous erysipelas of the face, beginning on the left side and moving towards the right, with pimples, vesicles; ecchymoses or petechia in exanthematous diseases; hæmorrhages in exanthematous diseases, small-pox, measles, scarlet fever, etc. Ulcers dark, bluish, bleeding profusely, sensitive to touch. Yellow, red and copper colored spots on the skin; purpura in large splotches, sensitive to touch. Miliary eruption soon turns livid or black, becomes vesicular, then pustulous and often gangrenous (Carbo veg., Ars., Carbol. acid. Crotalus). Septic poisoning from dissecting wounds; parts much swollen, purplish red or leaden hued, tongue dry, glossy, tremulous, < after sleep, all symptoms. Varicose veins ulcerate and discharge dark, watery, offensive fluid, very sensitive to touch. Bed sores in fevers that become dark, sensitive, inflamed, with black edges. Bluish colored pustules, with red streaks radiating from the lymphatics. Black, blue spots all over the body; carbuncles with rigors, nocturnal sweat, fever, prostration, great sensitiveness, discharge dark, bloody, or dark, with degenerated pus (Carbo veg.), attended with great burning, < after sleep and by bathing in cold water. Scarlatina maligna, advanced stages, typhoid states threatening gangrene.

Subjective—Itching all over the body in paroxysms, < at night, often changing to burning and stinging; very sensitive to weight of clothes. Ulcers, pustules, carbuncles, erysipelas, gangrene, with burning pains, chills, or chilly spells, followed by hot flashes in febrile diseases or at the menopause, malignancies appearing at that time.

Aggravation—Night, after sleep, contact, pressure, constriction, touch.

Amelioration—Cold bathing, (carbuncles, furuncles), while awake, open air.

Temperament—Bilious nervous.

LAMIUM ALBUM

Objective—Blisters on the heel, due to rubbing and pressure of the shoe, changing to a long-lasting, stubborn ulcer. Ulcers with swelling and redness of the surrounding part.

Subjective—Biting, pain as if excoriated, pricking, gnawing; itching of the arms and hands. Smarting, stinging and shooting.

LAPIS ALBUS

Objective—Carcinoma of the face, uterus, breasts. Affections of the glands and lymphatics; scrofulous affections; enlargement and indurations of the glands (Con., Iod., Kali iod.), especially the cervical; glandular tumors, goitre, lipoma, sarcoma, glandular and fibrous tumors, tubercular processes of the skin.

Subjective—Burning, shooting, stinging, pains in the breasts and uterus.

LACTIC ACID

Objective—Skin dry, hard, no sweat. Diabetes mellitus. Subjective—Profuse, offensive sweating of the feet (Sil., Baryta carb., Baryta iod., Iod., Psor.). Itching on various parts, redness on covered parts with slight burning and itching, > warmth, < cold, especially going quickly from warm to cold, or *vice versa*; itching and burning on going into cold air, followed by a creeping sensation in the affected part.

LEDUM PALUSTRE

Objective—Ledum is an anti-sycotic remedy adapted to a rheumatic and gouty diathesis (Coloc., Kalmia, Colch., Borac. ac., Ars., Benzoic ac., Mag. carb.); gouty concretions under the skin and in small joints; punctured wounds, injuries to the head, insect bites or bites of small, rabid animals. Papules or tubercles on the forehead and cheeks, as in brandy drinkers; black and blue places become green (Arn., Ham., Bellis per.) after injuries. Purple spots over the body like petechia. Purpura, erythema nodosum, scurfs on dry, small nodules, often renewed. Blood boils, urticaria, white but becoming red when rubbed, intense itching, stinging, burning. Stinging of wasps, bees, mosquitoes; punctured wounds, with sharp instruments (Hyp.). Eczema and acne of drunkards (Sulph. ac.).

Subjective—Discoloration still remains in contused parts, after pain and swelling has left. Skin hot, tense, hard in swellings. Dry skin, with violent itching, burning in open air. Sensation as of lice crawling on the surface in pruritus, < heat, night, motion. Pale, delicate, rheumatic or gouty patients who are always chilly.

Temperament—Motor.

LITHIUM CARBONICUM

Adapted to rheumatic and gouty patients, who suffer from kidney and bladder troubles. Urine scanty, dark, acrid with pain and tenesmus when passing; reddish brown, brick dust deposit (Lyc., Phos., Sep.). Skin rough as a grater, harsh, dry. Barber's itch, ringworm, circular furfuraceous patches on the skin. Skin of the whole body rough, dry; both cheeks covered with a thick crust.

Subjective—Itching and burning.

LYCOPODIUM

Objective—Blood boils; boils do not mature but remain blue; boils returning periodically; boils in the axillæ. Lupus, recent cases, shallow ulceration in pale, sallow patients. Large, jagged, pedunculated warts, exuding moisture and bleeding easily. Nevus maternus and vascular tumors. Eruption, first vesicular, then dry; humid, suppurating, full of deep rhagades, breeding lice, itching violently; intertrigo, raw places readily bleeding. Eczema on the face, genitals, legs, neck, fingers, hands; bleed easily and covered with thick crusts, with fetid secretion beneath. Moist, scald head, moist on and behind the ears. < right ear. Intertrigo between the thighs and labia,

18

forming flat, lard-like ulcers with inflamed edges. Ulcers bleed and burn when dressed; tearing, shooting, itching at night, burning when touched; fistulous, with hard, red edges, often shining and everted, with inflammatory swelling of the affected part. Cancerous ulcers, flat, with a bluish white base.

Scarlet fever, secondary eruption with dark, red blotches on the thighs, hands, back or face; during desquamation stage sudden rise of temperature, with weak pulse, hot, dry skin, scanty urine, with strangury, burning in the urethra, pain in the region of the kidneys; urine dark red, with brick dust sediment, containing albumen. Large, brown patches or macules on the face, bridge of nose or any part of the body in liver troubles (Sepia in uterine troubles). Herpes furfuraceous, yellow at base. and bleeding on face, in corners of the mouth; insensible, yellow brown, shrivelled herpes; herpes on the nape of neck, axillæ, thighs, calves of the legs. Psoriasis of the hands and fingers has the same furfuraceous look, occasionally fissured and bleeding. Freckles in large, brownish, coalescent patches. Pustules exuding bloody, corrosive, putrid pus, sometimes milky or curdled.

Eruptions about the knees, genitals, ears, face; glandular swellings, varicose veins on the legs, fissures on the heels with watery oozing.

Diseases.—Scarlet fever, measles, adenitis, alopecia, boils, chilblains, dandruff, erysipelas, ecthyma, eczema, erythema nodosum, lichen, nettle rash, chronic urticaria, freckles, goitre, herpes, intertrigo, arthritic nodosities, prurigo, scald head, scurvy, ulcers, warts, varices.

Subjective—Burning, or burning itching; itching as from fleas. Pricking, itching, corrosive itching, tingling itching, numb sensation in the parts affected. Pains drawing or tearing, shooting or stitching. Burning scalding itching, in eczema of the scalp, burning when touched.

Accompanying symptoms gastric disturbances, bloating in stomach and abdomen, belching of much gas, much commotion, rumbling of gas in stomach and abdomen.

Aggravation—Afternoon (4 P. M.); touch, pressure; right side; heat, wrapping up warm, wet or warm poultices, eating cabbage, oysters, wine, cold food.

Amelioration—Warm food and drinks, uncovering the head, loosing clothing.

As in the rule in other diseases, do not begin the treatment of a case of chronic skin trouble with Lycopodium; it, above all others, should follow some other remedy.

Temperament—Sang-mental.

LYSSIN

Objective—This remedy has been used very seldom in diseases of the skin, yet it was used by Hahnemann seventy years before Pasteur ever thought of it, and by many of Hahnemann's followers in many forms of mania, puerperal mania, especially, as well as in rabies. In 1885 the author cured a case of puerperal mania of the worst form with Lyssin 6 potency, as he then was not familiar with the higher potencies; in fact, they were then almost unknown in this country.

Symptoms—Paroxysms of intense coldness, with pain in the spine soon after being bitten. Bluish discoloration of the bitten part (Lach.). Pustules about the affected part, red spots in a circle; scar red for a long time, after bite occasionally it would break open. Malignant ulcer from the bite. Cancerous sores. Herpes circinatus appeared after the bite of a rabid dog. Bites from rabid animals as well as the dog.

Subjective—Biting, itching, < scratching; quick tendency of the wound to heal (leprosy); great blueness of the veins in the affected part. Slightest touch brings on convulsions (Stram.). Pain in the bitten part burning, and extended over the whole body; felt very strangely, sensations of pricking, boring, burning in the bitten part, yet in some cases there was no pain. Shock-like sensations down the arm and fingers. Great sensitiveness to a draft of air. Nervous twitchings and trembling of the whole body; the sight or sound of running water aggravates all complaints. *Fear of becoming mad.* Saliva tough, ropy, viscid, frothy, greatly increased; spasm of the esophagus on swallowing water: bites, snarls, growls at attendant.

Aggravation—Bright light, running water, drinking, riding in a carriage, touch, draft of air (cold).

MAGNESIA CARB

Objective—Small, red, elevated, smooth herpes, scaling off, on calves of legs, chest and about the mouth (about the mouth, Hep., Nat. mur., Aco., Rhus, Mer. viv., Sep., Puls., Bry., Ars.). Nodes under the skin (gouty.) Psoriasis or pityriasis on palmar surfaces. Tubercles on the wrists pouring out clear water when pressed.

Subjective—Itching and dryness of the skin; itching, < scratching; vesicles after scratching. Painful, small, red, herpes, scaling off. Sour smell of the whole body, sycotic child (Rheum, Mag. mur.).

Aggravation—Evening, in bed. Milk, during menses.
Amelioration—In open air, if warm weather (Puls).
Temperament—Sang-motive.

MAGNETIS ARCTICUS

Objective—Red eruption in palms of the hands. Felons, herpes, itch-like pustules, deep, lentil-sized ulcers.

Subjective—Burning or burning tearing in the skin, pricking in the soles of the feet in small spots, tingling

itching, hot creepy sensation in affected parts; pricking
from knees to feet. Crawling all over the skin; herpes
with burning pains, excessive weariness of the lower
extremities, < walking.

MAGNETIS AUSTRALIS

Objective—Felons, with painful drawing, darting,
jerking, stinging, burning (Apis). Ingrowing toe nails
which penetrate the flesh (Sil.), with above pains; usually
the great toe is affected. Many cures reported, with no
return. (It works best in potencies above the 1 m.).

Subjective—Itching, stinging, tearing here and there.
Symptoms greatly aggravated by change of weather
from dry to wet (similar to Rhus in that respect). Corrosive itching, lancinating, pulsating pains at root of nails
(Hep., pulsating in suppuration). Mental symptoms, des-
pondency, discouraged, easily angered, irritable and
cross. Suppuration scanty.

MANGANUM

Objective—Itching herpes; rhagades in the bends of
the knees, or on the skin, < sweating. Chronic suppuration of the skin, especially about the joints. Lepra vulgaris, psoriasis, pityriasis. Malignant ulcer with blue border, following a scratch of the nail. Psoriasis with
white, shiny, hard, adherent scales.

Subjective—Itching in hollow of knee, in the palms;
burning in small, red spots on the chest. Pityriasis rubra,
scales in great quantities thrown off, exposing a red, dry
surface. Lichen, itching, < night, ceases when scratching.

MEDORRHINUM

Objective—Gonorrhea or for the constitutional effects

of bad treatment, suppressions and diseases arising out of them; sycotic diseases, rheumatism, gout, warts, moles, pelvic inflammations, acne and all skin eruptions arising from the gonorrheal taint. Malignant growths can often be traced to gonorrhea, and they may be arrested or much benefited by this remdey. It bears the same relation to sycosis as Psorinum does to psora or Syphilinum does to syphilis. Mental symptoms are valuable, forgets words, names, sentences, has to ask the name of his most intimate friend, anxious about his condition, fears the physician will not take his case right, repeats his symptoms, is very peevish, freful, impatient. Face much paler, greenish yellow appearance of the face, blotches and pimples on the face, large, angry looking acne on the face during or after the menses, in young girls with the gonorrheal taint. Face covered with acne, and accompanied with a greasy appearance of the face (Mer.). Gonorrheal flow thin, mixed with opaque, whitish mucus. Stains linen yellow, meatus swollen, puffy, drawing and burning when urinating, or thin, mucous, gleety discharge with soreness of the urethra. Great yellowishness of the skin. Small, pedunculated warts on various parts of the body (Staph., Bell., Thuja). Warts of the filiform variety appear profusely scattered over the trunk or on covered parts, often within forty-eight hours after giving the remedy; constitutional symptoms all relieved or much benefited. Acute eruption of warts after suppressed gonorrhea. Reproduced gonorrheal flow with or without appearance of warts; red moles, spider spots on the body, especially on the face; nevis dark, velvety, red, accompanied with warts.

Subjective—Oozing from the rectum or vagina of a thin, watery fluid, which smells like fish brine, musty or stale fish odor, which excoriates, producing a dark red erythema (Kreos., Ars., Carbol. ac., Sulph.). Itching red spots on the skin, < undressing. Dryness and burning in the nostrils, stuffy, stopped up feeling in young infants and children. Sensations as if icy cold insects on the skin, intense burning and itching in the palms, intense, unbearable itching in vagina, labia, rectum, due to corrosive discharges; pruritus ani, drives him almost to the verge of insanity, not relieved by suppositories of Opium or Cocaine. Ulcers, pustules, excoriations discharging a greenish, yellowish, dirty, water-like fluid, which smells rank, putrid, musty or like stale fish, excoriating parts passed over. Umbilicus discharges for months after birth, same characteristic odor, color and consistency. Itching worse thinking of it; great heat and soreness after scratching.

Aggravation— < thinking about the disease; winter, from 10 to 11 A.M.

Amelioration—Lying on stomach (Puls.); dry weather.

MERCURIUS

Objective—Mercurius is an anti-syphilitic as well as an anti-psoric. Skin yellow, in icterus, with biting over abdomen.

Erythema, upon which vesicles, form and pour out a thin, clear fluid, vesicles quickly broken, contents dessicate, redness remains for a week or longer; round spots shining through the skin of a coppery color. Small, flat, red blotches on the sexual parts, chest, abdomen and inner side of thighs. Scurfy eruption beginning on head and spreading over the whole body; dry, rash-like, readily bleeding eruption. Desquamation all over, < on hands and feet. Miliary papules in circular groups, raised, rough, bright red, irritable, itching, < at night. Eczema, developing small, superficial, moist ulcers; eczema with yellow crusts and inflamed surroundings. Herpes burning when touched, humid, with large scales on the edges, moist vesicles surrounded by dry scales, easily bleeding. Very small, transparent vesicles, containing a watery fluid. Herpetic spots and suppurating pustules sometimes running together, forming dry, scaly spots, or crusts with acrid discharges. Herpes zoster girdling from back to abdomen, attended with burning pains and gastric disturbances, tendency to suppurate. Intertrigo raw, bloody discharge, tendency to ulcerate, < at night. Small pimples or vesicles change to ulcers; impetigo, pustules have a tendency to ulcerate; base of pustule very red or inflamed. Eczema, yellowish crusts bleeding easily, red, raised, humid eruption; fetid, putrid ulcers on legs, ulcers discharging an acrid, excoriating ichor; spongy, bluish, readily bleeding ulcer. Secondary syphilitic eruptions, all forms. Ulcers large, bleeding, margins everted like raw meat, their bases covered with a caseous coat. Carious ulcers, exostosis, gouty swellings, glandular swellings, with or without suppuration. Cold swellings, slowly suppurating abscesses. Chancre, gonorrhea, blennorrhagia, urethritis and vaginitis.

Subjective—Itching of the whole body, < at night when getting warm; itching that became pleasant on scratching; violent itching, < night; intolerable sticking itching, as from flea bites. Itching all over the body, with nettle rash, > by cold and < night, in bed, from warmth. In syphilitic eruptions as well as in many other cases Mercury has no pain or itching. Itching eruptions with burning after scratching. Itching intolerable when he gets warm at his work. Dry, elevated, burning itching tetter on the whole body, especially on the arms, wrists, legs, hands, between fingers, (eczema); itching so great in bed has to uncover or find a cool place (like Sulphur), or gets out of bed in order to get relief, Scarlatina, burning heat, face very red and swollen, thirst, restlessness, > uncovering and getting cool, fright and starting during sleep, delirium, sensorial depression and sopor, great oppression of the chest, short, quick respiration, anxiety before the appearance of the eruption. Mercury patients dread the night in all diseases. Tongue foul coated, flabby, thick, white or yellow pasty coating, tongue shows the imprint of the teeth; taste metallic; putrid odor from the mouth, breath foul, offensive; saliva increased, ropy, viscid, tenacious. Pains, < at night and before a storm in chronic cases.

Aggravation—Night, approach of night; heat of bed, covering up warm, perspiring, wet or stormy weather, touch, scratching.

Amelioration—Cold, cool air, dry weather, daytime; rest in bed.

Best adapted to light haired persons, with lax muscles and skin.

Temperament—Sang-ment-vital.

MERCURIUS CORROSIVUS

Objective—Severe, stubborn forms of eczema, when the Mercurius vivus seems to be indicated but does not relieve. Ulcers very red and deep, greatly aggravated at night, discharging an ichorous, corrosive discharge. Small-pox with intense inflammation and ulceration of the throat. Ulcers that perforate and become phagedenic; scorbutic spots over the whole body, mingled with itch-like eruptions, herpes and boils.

Subjective—Burning and redness of the skin, with formation of small vesicles. Burning and stinging heat in skin, cannot rest anywhere for heat. Sweats profusely at night; skin cold and clammy, perspiration fetid.

Temperament—Sang-ment-vital.

MERCURIUS IODATUS FLAVUS

Subjective—Troublesome itching all over the body, $<$ at night. Itching, pricking over the body, $<$ night. Itching accompanied with a fine, bright red eruption on the chest and abdomen. Painless chancres with swelling of the inguinal glands. Glands swollen, hard, indurated (Iod., Con., Mer. protoiod.). Itching not $>$ by scratching. Pains throbbing boring, cramp-like. This remedy follows Lachesis in scarlatina. Crusta lactea with dry crusts and intolerable itching at night.

MERCURIUS IODATUS RUBER

Objective—Hard fissures and cracks; very deep crack in the centre of the lip (Kali iod.); hard papules here and there; pustules, with an inflamed base, sore to touch, itching slightly. Syphilitic ulcers, diphtheritic looking ulcers, dark red with much inflammation. Indurated Hunterian chancre. Bubo discharging for a year; old scrofulous, syphilitic ulcers, spreading syphilitic eruptions all over the body, moist offensive smelling ulcers. Scarlatina, large, flat, angry looking ulcers in the throat, tonsils covered with a fetid diphtheritic exudate. Lupus and condylomata.

MEZEREUM

Objective—Light haired persons of phlegmatic temperament. Skin wrinkled and in folds. Brownish miliary rash on chest, arms, thighs, red, itching rash on head and over the whole body, violent itching rash on nape of neck, back and thighs. Itching eruption after vaccination. Scurf-like fish scales on back, chest, thighs and scalp. Crusts thick, lamellated like rupia, bloody secretion beneath. Distressing exanthema, burning at night, compelled to scratch until the epidermis is removed and the denuded part is covered with a crust. Eczema, itching intolerably, copious serous exudation; herpes zoster with severe neuralgia pains, itching, after scratching turns into burning, < in bed, from touch, vesicles turn into brownish crusts. Vesicles appear around ulcers, itch violently and burn like fire, vesicles dry up, leaving crusts. The whole skin covered with elevated white crusts; head covered with thick, leather-like crusts, under which thick, white pus collects, hair glued and matted together, pus often ichorous, offensive, breeding vermin. Ulcers, with thick, yellowish white crusts, under which thick, yellow pus collects.

Subjective—Violent itching, < in bed, from touch, burning and changing place after scratching. Eczema, with intolerable itching and copious exudation; during violent itching and burning complains of chilliness, feeling of coldness along the spine and extremities. Pruritus senilis. Child continually scratches the face in eczema, which is covered with blood; face and forehead hot and red, child restless, irritable, itching, < at night, tears off the crusts, ichor from scratched surface excoriates. Moist itching eruption on the head and behind the ears. Eruption on scalp preceded by headache, scalp covered with scurf, hair comes out in handfuls, eyebrows and eyelashes drop out, scalp and face itch violently, < getting warm. Dry eruption on scalp with intolerable itching, as if head was an ants' nest. Itching and biting on the margin of the lids. Blepharitis. Eczema of the lids with hard, thick crusts, exuding pus.

Aggravation—Evening, night, when touched.

Amelioration—Open air.

Temperament—Sang-lymphatic.

MURIATIC ACID

Objective—Face, heat of face; glowing red cheeks in scarlet fever (Bell.). Sudden reddening of the face with coma (scarlet fever); red, itching pimples on the forehead, cheeks, around the mouth, whole face red, every summer (eczema solaris). Ulcers painful, deep, putrid, covered with scurf, more frequently on lower extremities. Malignant small-pox, with the low typhoid state peculiar to this remedy. Scarlet fever, erysipelas, bluish color of the skin (Carbo veg.); petechia, hæmorrhages from internal organs, sliding down in bed, patients with dark hair, eyes and complexion.

Subjective—Burning at edge of ulcers, itching, stinging in skin.

Temperament—Bil-motive.

NATRUM ARSENICUM

Objective—Corners of the mouth fissured, also indurated (Nit. ac., Pet., Nat. mur., Tub.). Squamous eruption, scales thin, white, and when removed leave the skin slightly reddened; itch, < when warm or from exercise.

Temperament—Bil-motor.

NATRUM CARBONICUM

Objective—Skin of whole body becomes dry, rough and cracked in places.

Red vesicles filled with fluid in bend of elbow, in fold between genitals and thigh, also on the chin. Spreading and suppurating herpes; herpes iris suppurating. Yellow rings like the remains of herpes; freckles on the face dark brown. Warts ulcerate, sensitive to touch. Rose colored blotches in leprous patients, ulcerating tubercles of the face and other parts of the body.

Subjective—Burning in injured parts, with shooting and incisive pains. Itching as from fleas, tingling.

Temperament—Bil-motive.

NATRUM MURIATICUM

Objective—Skin yellowish color, delicate, dirty looking, dry, withered, irritable; great rawness and soreness of the skin in intertrigo. Small, white vesicles with clear, watery contents, which burst, leaving a thin scurf. Herpes about the mouth and on the arms, thighs, humid on the scrotum and thighs, during fevers, in the bends of the elbows and knees, moist oozing. Herpes circinatus, pemphigus, blisters appearing on red, burning spots, with clear, watery contents, watery blebs. Herpes zoster; rupia; blisters, not pustular. Nettle rash over whole body, large, red blotches, with violent itching, after violent exercise. Chronic urticaria. Miliary eruption all over the body. Acne punctata. Comedones, eczema, raw and inflamed, scurfy and discharging a corrosive fluid, < in edges of the hair, on genitals; tetter in bends of the joints oozing an acrid fluid; crusts with deep cracks, scaly eruptions on flexor surfaces. Eczema from eating too much salt. Superficial ulcers, red, angry, smarting, surrounded by vesicles, no suppuration. Boils, blood boils, warts in the palms of hands. Infantile marasmus, from defective nourishment; child has an old look (Mer., Sulph., Psor.). Face oily, shiny, as if greased. Eczema that appears in the vesicular form, beginning as small transparent vesicles that appear after scratching, seldom forming pustules or suppurating; but forming thin, dry crusts and desquamating.

Subjective—Dry eczema, beginning by intense itching, with no eruption, very small, white vesicles form after scratching, which dry up when broken into dry, scaly crusts; itching, < in the evening when undressing, a constant symptom, pale, active, thin people who crave salt. Itching, > by scratching, whole body is torn and full of superficial scratch marks, skin pale, hands and feet cold. Skin dry, rough, scurvy-like; itching, > by scratching.

18

When the little vesicles are broken, they sometimes show a tendency to suppurate, but only a faint show of pus is present. Itching < behind ears, bends of knees, elbows, border of hair and scalp, < 10 A. M. or in evening, cool air or undressing. Itching, pricking, stinging, gnawing, shooting. Great rawness and smarting in intertrigo, skin troubles and pruritus, < during the full moon (Clematis).

Diseases—Acne punctata, boils, corns, eczema, felons, goitre, herpes, herpes circinatus, herpes zoster, nettle rash, chronic hives, scrofulosis, tubercular and latent syphilitic patients, varices, warts.

Aggravation—Evening, undressing, marked periodicity in many diseases, violent exercise (reverse, Sepia).

Amelioration—Fasting, open air, perspiring.

Temperament—Bil-motor.

NATRUM SULPHURICUM

Objective—Diseases induced by damp weather or living in damp houses (Rhus); patient feels every change of weather, especially from dry to wet (Rhus). Every spring skin affections appear (Graph., Psor.). It is a true anti-sycotic. Vesicles and pimples on the face, smooth erysipelas of the face, vesicles on the lower lip, vesicular eruption around the mouth (Ars., Nat. mur., Rhus, Hep.). Fistulous abscesses of years' standing, discharging watery pus, surrounded by a broad, blue line, burrowing. Eczema moist and oozing profusely. Moist skin affections with bilious symptoms, edematous inflammation of the skin. Erysipelas smooth, red, shiny (Bell.); tingling and painful swelling, sycotic excrescences, wartlike, red lumps all over the body. Small, itching crusts between the scrotum and thighs, scalp, neck, chest; > scratching. Red, knotty lumps on head above the ears, on the forehead and left side of nape of neck. Brown spots on the inner surface of both thighs after syphilis. Water blisters on fingers, especially on the dorsum of fingers, blisters filled with clear water, chronic suppuration about finger nails, palms sore and raw, and exude a watery fluid. Paronychia, patient pale and feeble, heavy feeling in the head, loss of appetite, in the evening chills and heat, after a blister, filled with water, which came on the last phalanx, nail swollen all around, very red, painful (Hep., Sil., Mag., Aust.); yellow pus around the root of nail, pain, > out of doors, than in a warm room (Puls.). Inflammation and suppuration about the nails, pustules on the palms of hands, fingers, wrists, single, widely scattered, very little suppuration, cracks and fissures on the fingers, hands, wrists, bleeding slightly, < in the spring, full moon, damp weather, hands stiff, dry, hot, cannot bend them without inducing pain.

Subjective—Burning of the soles of feet, extending to knees (Phos., Opium); eruption very sore and sensitive, shooting, piercing pain in pustules.

Aggravation—Dampness, wet weather, undressing, < (Nat. mur., Hep., Psor., Ars., Sil.).

Amelioration—Pressure with the hand, dry weather, after breakfast (Nux vom.).

Temperament—Bil-motive.

NICCOLUM

Subjective—Itching all over body, but < on neck, as from fleas, not > by scratching, but followed by small vesicles (Nat. mur.). Fine burning, stinging, biting, as from bees (Apis). Small tubercles after scratching. Itching, on face, at anus, scrotum. Burning in the eyes, face, tip of nose, anus.

Aggravation—Evening and at night.

Amelioration—Open air.

NITRIC ACID

Objective—Phagedenic blisters on toes, scabby, moist, itching, offensive eruption, paining as from splinters when touched (Hep.). Humid, stinging eruption on vertex and temples; also, in beard; bleeding easily when scratched and feeling very sore when lain on. Single, burning, moist sores on scalp (syphilis). Small warts on lids (upper). Warts on upper lip, smarts and bleeds on washing, painful to touch; large, jagged, often pedunculated, exuding moisture and bleeding easily, condylomata, elevated exuberant, cock's-comb or cauliflower-like growths, moist, discharging a thin, greenish, yellow or bloody, fetid discharge (Kali iod., Kreo).

Syphilitic eruptions, in secondary or tertiary stages, with superficial ulcers, and bone pains. Ulcers bleed when touched, shooting, splinter-like pains, edges hard, everted, irregular, exuberant, granulations, tendency to fungus growth, carious, mercurial or syphilitic. Painful chilblains, corns, warts, herpes. Rhagades, deep, bleeding (Graph., Kali iod.). Osteo-nodes, with sticking, shooting pains at night. Offensive night sweats, with dark, strong smelling urine, purpura, or purpura hæmorrhagica in exanthematous diseases, blood bright red, not clotted, tongue dry, deep velvety red, urine offensive, burning, pungent skin, irregular, quick, hard pulse, prostration, delirium or listlessness, great weakness and trembling, in low forms of fever. In-grown toe nails with splinter-like pains, foul smelling foot sweat (Baryta c., Sil., Psor., Mag. aust.). Cancer, with profuse bleeding; bleeding as soon as touched, sticking pains, sloughing and undermining of the ulcer; ulcer flat, with elevated zig-zag edges, painless or painful, looking like raw meat; spongy, bloody, copious, thin discharge, bleed when touched.

Subjective—Burning, itching, stinging, shooting, lancinating, splinter-like pains in ulcers, < at night. Discharges thin acrid, offensive, of a brownish or dirty yellow color.

Aggravation—Night, touch, during perspiration, walking.

Amelioration—Open air, when riding in a carriage.

Temperament—Bil-motor.

NUX VOMICA

Objective—Skin diseases induced by over-eating. Beer, wine or whisky drinkers (Ledum, brandy drinkers). Irritable, impatient, intemperate people, who when sick are hard to get along with. Urticaria induced by eating fats, rich pastry or much meat (Puls., fat foods; Ars., cold foods), late suppers, etc. Acne or papillary eruptions following over-eating, cheese eating or rich foods, constipation or errors in diet. Gouty conditions from the same causes. Irritable, morose, quarrelsome, easily angered, before or after bilious attacks. Nux antidotes the bad effects of drugs, or eruptions induced by many of the vegetable compounds. Skin sallow in liver or stomach troubles, sensitive and sore to touch. Tendency to boils with gastric derangements that are very sore and sensitive; should be frequently given in place of Arnica or Hepar; there is usually a very little tendency to suppurate; tongue coated dirty brown, bad taste in mouth, patient cross, irritable, with temporal headaches, chilly, > by heat and by being quiet and lone, sleepy, drowsy in the evening or after eating.

Subjective—Burning, pricking like flea bites. Eruptions sore and painful. Skin sensitive or sore. Terrible pricking, stinging, itching; itching of icterus < in the evening and by cold.

Aggravation—Evening, after eating, cold, before breakfast, contact. Mental worry, noise, over-eating, rich food, spices, narcotics, spirituous liquors, when constipated.

Amelioration—Quiet, alone. Warmth, external heat, sleep; also, > as the day proceeds.

Temperament—Bil-motor.

OPIUM

Objective—Red blotches after scratching. Chilblains on fingers and toes; the whole body looks red or blue and cyanotic, face blue, congested, blue spots in scarlet fever, burning heat, soporous stupor, coma. Sudden retrocession of eruptions with convulsions or paralysis of the brain. Suppurations and ulcerations usually painless. Skin looks dry, wrinkled, in marasmus of children. Acne rosacea in drunkards or Opium eaters, parts red, flushed, bloated, livid, swollen.

Subjective—Burning heat in scarlet fever with stupor, very troublesome itching, fine pricking, desire to uncover, feet and hands burn like fire (Sulph., Phos., Sang.). Boils, papules, pimples, on the face, neck chest, very red or dark blue, and not sensitive.

Aggravation—Covering, getting heated, during and after sleep.

Amelioration—Cold, constant walking.

Temperament—Sang-lymphatic.

OXALIC ACID

Objective—Face pale and livid, often with sunken eyes. face covered with cold sweat, fingers and nails livid, heaviness of the fingers, skin mottled, eruption in circular patches, warts, ringworm, corns, tinea barbara.

Subjective—Exceeding sensitive skin, with vesicular eruption, < from sweating itching on neck and fingers, smarting and soreness in the skin, < on the face, sweating, shaving.

PALLADIUM

Spots, like flea bites, above the lips or on the right side of nose; small elevations here and there like nettle rash; red on a white base, whiter than the surrounding skin, warts on the knuckles.

Subjective—Itching, crawling, as from fleas, > from scratching, but appears in some other place. Burning, itching on face and left groin, itching on inner side of left ankle, pustules under eyebrows burn and bite, < rubbing, > scratching.

PETROLEUM

Blisters on the heels, blotches on the calves of both legs. Tubercular changes in the lymphatic glands with previous history of skin eruptions. Moist eczema on the scalp, behind the ears, on the hands, in light haired, irritable, quarrelsome people; nearly the whole head covered with thick, yellow eczematous crusts, hair glued together by the exudation, itching intense, scratching induces bleeding. *Thick, greenish yellow crusts, burning and itching, redness, rawness cracks bleed easily, thick, yellowish exudations.* Skin around the eyes dry and scurfy (Nat. mur.). Scurfs around the mouth, papular eruption at corner of mouth. Whole skin of body sore and painful, unhealthy, even slight wounds suppurate and spread, general tendency to fester, slow to heal. Rhagades. < in winter (Graph., Tub., Kali sulph., Psor.); hands chap, crack, burn and itch intolerably, itching, sore, moist surfaces or deep cracks; cracks behind the ears; face lips, oozing moisture. Vesicular eruption forming thick crusts, oozing pus, skin harsh, dry, deep cracks and fissures which bleed and suppurate. Itching herpes followed by ulcers. Itching burning pustules, with great lassitude, < in fresh air. Boils, fissures, tinea favosa, burns, scalds.

Herpetic eruption on scrotum, exuding moisture, skin dry, cracked and bleeding; sweat and moisture on external genitals of both sexes.

Subjective—Painful itching, chilblains, burning like fire, moist oozing < in cold weather. Heat and burning of the soles of the feet, foul smelling perspiration of the feet, pustules itch and burn. Itching sore, moist eruptions with chills. Burning, itching in corns.

Aggravation—< in winter, riding in a carriage, morning.

Temperament—Sang-motive.

PHOSPHORUS

Subjective—Adapted to *tall, slender* persons of sanguine temperament, tubercular taint, fair, delicate skin, blonde or red hair, soft, silken eye lashes. Herpes dry or humid, squamous. Erysipelas upon the arms, occiput and nape of neck, bluish red in appearance. Variola in typhoid cases when the pustules do not fill with pus, but degenerate into largs blisters. Abscesses and indurations of the mammæ, copious bleeding from small wounds, purpura hæmorrhagica in exanthematous diseases, blood pours from bleeding surfaces. Psoriasis on the knees, elbows, legs and eyebrows. Pityriasis, brown spots on the skin, or yellow blotches on the abdomen or chest, red, sanguinous spots, petechia, purpura, ecchymosis. Dry, scaly skin, desquamation, or dry furfuraceous herpes. All the eruptions of Phosphorus, like Sulphur or Nat. mur., are usually dry. Pemphigus, painful, hard blisters, full to bursting, no itching. Urticaria, hands, arms and body covered with itching blotches. Sore, excoriated spots on the skin, rhagades. Phlegmonous inflammation, chronic or suppurating, openings with hectic fever; ulcers, often with caries. Fistulous ulcers with high edges, exuberant granulations, purulent discharge, thin and ichorous, erysipelatous blush often radiating around the ulcer, burning and stinging pains, hectic fever, with night sweats and cough and diarrhea. Open cancers and polypi bleed readily, fungus hematodes. Leprosy, later stages, brown spots on tubercles; tubercles on the trunk or buttocks, discolored borders around white spots. Scarlatina with suddenly repelled rash, followed by lung or chest symptoms, in tubercular patients. Sometimes hæmorrhages or brain symptoms develop in severe cases. Measles followed by pneumonia, cough, hectic conditions and general involvement of the lungs. Variola with bloody pustules, hæmorrhages ·or lung complications.

Aggravation—Evening, before midnight (reverse, Ars.); heat or cold in extremes.

Amelioration—In the dark, cold or cold food until it becomes warm.

Temperament—Bil-mental.

PHYTOLACCA

Objective—Barber's itch, chronic cases when Sulphur failed to help. (Barber's itch is a form of sycosis, therefore it requires an anti-sycotic remedy to cure it.) Tinea capitis, eczema capitis, eczema of the scalp in sycotic or gouty patients. Squamous eruptions, pityriasis, psoriasis, ringworm, herpes circinatus, lichen, lupus, ulcers, gouty conditions in the skin and the joints, warts, whitlow, syphilitic sores, scarlatina, measles.

Very ugly, black-looking, tettery eruption, blackness looks like gangrene, boils, disposition to boils, especially near ulcers (Hepar papules), painful, on the back, behind the ears. Ulcers looking as if punched out, lardaceous base, pus watery, fetid, ichorous, shooting, lancinating, jerking pains, syphilitic or cancerous ulcers of the breast. Scirrhus of the mammæ, cancer of the legs and of the face, Erythematous blotches, irregular, slightly raised, pale red, ending in dark red or purple spots. Scarlatina, high fever, headache, both sides of the throat covered with membrane, grayish in color, with rash on the body. Eruption dry, of a shrivelled appearance, in passing hand over skin it feels like brown paper; urine suppressed, hands and feet burning hot, cannot keep them covered (Sulph., Phos.); restless, tongue dry in the centre, sides coated brown, diphtheria or scarlet fever.

Drawing in cicatrices, rheumatic, neuralgic pains, rheumatic or syphilitic inflammations of the fibrous tissue, sheaths of nerves, periosteum, glands inflamed, swollen, indurated, gonorrheal buboes, epididymitis and other inflammatory glandular swellings. Pus watery, sanious, fetid, ichorous.

Subjective—Pains in long bones, nerve sheaths, periosteum, syphilitic pains in periosteum and bones, joints, < from midnight until morning, < motion, contact, damp weather. Pains sharp, cutting, burning, aching, < damp weather, pains like electric shocks, shooting, shifting rapidly (Ferr. phos.) follows Rhus tox.

Aggravation—Damp weather, rainy weather, midnight until morning, cold.

Amelioration—Warmth, dry weather, rest.

Temperament—Bil-motive.

PIX LIQUIDA

Objective—Tubercular subjects, in the third stage of phthisis, tubercles break down and discharge a purulent matter. Eczema on the backs of the hands, itching intolerable at night, bleeding when scratched.

Subjective—Skin cracked, bleeding when scratched, intolerable itching at night, with sleeplessness, often a pain in the third left costal cartilage, proving very imperfect; has suppressed many eruptions, especially eczema.

PLANTAGO MAJOR

Objective—Vesicles on the hands with swelling and redness. Papules which exude a yellowish humor and form crusts, erythema, burns, Rhus tox. poisoning, hands and face red, swollen, covered with vesicles, itching violently. Inflammations of the skin involving cellular tissue. Dry, scaly eruption on lower lip, erysipelas of mammæ.

Subjective—Burning after rubbing and when scratched, violent itching in erysipelas and Rhus poisoning, with vesication. Pricking, stinging pains, shooting pains, marked inflammation in incised wounds, glands, bruises, frost bites, chilblains, bites of animals.

PLUMBUM METALLICUM

Objective—Skin rough, dry, scaly, yellowish, pale, clay-colored and dingy. Serous infiltration and puffy appearance of the skin. Burns when there are yellowish, ichorous vesicles, burning itching and threatening gangrene. Burning in ulcers, small wounds become easily inflamed and suppurate, indurations after inflammation. Gout of great toe or of thumb, numb feeling in the part, obstinate constipation in most diseases.

Subjective—Numbness in the part affected, pains very severe, paroxysmal, colicky, $>$ by pressure, $<$ night and evening. Burning in ulcers. Face greasy, shiny, blue line on margin of gums.

Aggravation—Night, evening.

Amelioration—Rubbing, hard pressure.

Temperament—Bil-motive.

PSORINUM

Objective—This remedy is to be grouped with such remedies as Sulph., Syph., Medorrh., Tub.; it stands side by side in value. It reaches down deeply into the life forces, covering every organ, every tissue, as well as the mental sphere. The psoric patient is full of fears, always despairing, never going to get better. They are extremely sensitive to cold, all the excretions are offensive, the whole body has a filthy smell. They are always hungry, > by eating. The skin is dry, scaly or moist, fetid, suppurating eruptions, oozing a sticky, offensive fluid (Graph.), from behind the ears, etc. Suppressed eruption (Sulph.). The hair is dry, lustreless, tangles easily, glues together; averse to having the head uncovered (Sil.). Scurfy eruptions in children, large, yellow vesicles around and between the crusts. Profusely suppurating, fetid eruption on the head, with rawness and soreness behind the ears (Pet., Hep.). Large humid blotches on the head, with scabby eruptions on the face. Pustules and boils on the head, with copious flow of pus. Child scratches until the blood flows. Humid, scabby eruption on the head, foul smelling, full of lice, glandular swellings. The eruptions of this remedy may either be dry or moist, squamæ in patches, scales pile up half an inch on the scalp or in patches on the body, dry or moist and bad smelling; scales large, thin, flaky, constantly desquamating, red and angry beneath with oozing, or dry, scaly, dark red, scrofulous inflammations of the margins of the lids, eyelids inflamed, puffy, child constantly rubbing them; thick crusts form on the margin of the lids, or bran-like tetter (Ars., Sulph., Mer., Bar. iod., Tub., Graph., Syph.); eruption covered the whole face of a child, moist, offensive smelling eruption. Moist crusts behind the ears, cheeks, corners of the mouth.

Eruptions in the bends of elbows and around wrists, whole surface has a dirty, dingy look (Sulph.), as if the patient had never washed; excessive secretion of the sebaceous glands (Mer., Hep., Mezer., Sulph.). Fine, dry eruption disappearing by desquamation, Psoriasis, dark red or brownish color, scales thick, grayish white; patient dreads the cold, yet itching is < in warm room or in bed. Ulcers, deep, penetrating, ichorous, on the face and legs, old, with fetid pus, violently itching, scrofulous, with swelling of the bones. Moist, itching condylomata.

Subjective—Much itching, tawny, dirty colored skin. Thick, dirty looking mass, composed of scales and pus, itching intensely. Burning stinging itching, sleepless from intolerable itching (Sulph.), stings when body becomes warm, < night when in bed (Sulph.). Scratches until it bleeds, itching with burning or with a biting sensation, < in cool air, night, in bed. Burning itching pustules after vaccination.

Aggravation—Night, in bed, cold air, undressing, suppressed eruptions.

Amelioration—Perspiring, warmth, eating, summer.

PULSATILLA

Subjective—Indicated in light or sandy hair, blue-eyed, mild and timid disposition, women more especially. Urticaria, with diarrhea; itching, < at night, from pastry, fat food, delayed menses. Erysipelas, passive form, spreads rapidly, bluish color, thirstless, low forms of fever, Chilblains, with bluish red swelling and rhagades. Pimply eruptions on different parts of the body; moles or freckles on young girls (Sep., Fer.). Measles, catarrhal symptoms very prominent (Euph.); coryza and profuse lachrymation; cough usually dry at night and loose by day. After scarlet fever, pain in the ears and deafness; varices in pregnant women, highly inflamed. Ulcers bleed easily, burn, itch and sting around their borders which are hard or red, fistulous, < in the afternoon or evening, burning like hot coals in the ulcer, > by cool air or cool bathing; discharge profuse, greenish yellow pus. Wounds suppurate; pus thick, bland, profuse, < in warm room, > in the open air and by cold bathing. Acne in young girls, < at or before menses, with a tendency to form pustules, containing greenish yellow pus, > by cold bathing. In the skin as in other diseases the symptoms are passive, changeable, discharges profuse (sycotic pus). Abscess; bleeding readily, stinging and cutting pains, bluish red swelling surrounding the parts; pus bloody or yellowish green, copious; pain in abscesses as from subcutaneous ulceration. Pains and other symptoms often accompanied with chilliness, yet feels < in a warm room. Affections of mucous surfaces, pus profuse, thick, yellowish green, bland. Itching not marked.

Aggravation—Warm room, afternoon, evening, warm applications, warm water, ulcers.

Amelioration—Close, warm room, cool bathing, motion, walking slowly about, open air.

Temperament—Sang-phlegmatic.

RANUNCULUS BULBOSUS

Objective—Blisters between the fingers emitting a thin, yellow fluid, dark blue vesicles emitting a dark, yellow lymph, and covered with a horny, herpetic scurf. Flat, corrosive ulcers, with sharp edges. Herpetic or vesicular eruption with intolerable itching; vesicular eruption as from burns.

Herpes zoster, vesicles filled with a yellowish serum

(Rhus tox.), which burn; vesicles sometimes dark, followed with sharp, stitching pains. Pemphigus, blisters very large, burst, leaving raw surfaces; in children blisters from two to three inches in diameter, restlessness and prostration, constantly returning eruptions of blisters, secreting a foul-smelling, gluey matter, forming crusts and healing from the centre. Eczema, vesicular, followed by scurfs, then a fresh eruption of vesicles, with burning and itching, attended by thickening of the skin and the formation of hard, horny crusts. Shingles with intercostal neuralgia. Flat, burning, stinging ulcers, with ichorous discharge; pus sanious or acrid.

Subjective—Burning stinging in ulcers, intolerable burning, itching in vesicles and herpes. Herpes with neuralgia (intercostal); crawling, creeping, itching in scalp and palms of hands and fingers.

Aggravation—Morning and evening, contact, on entering a cool place, wet weather (Rhus).

Temperament—Nervo-bilious. Ranunculus scler, symptoms quite similar to the bulbosus.

RHUS TOX

Objective—Rhus tox, the true anti-sycotic. Every expression of this great remedy's action is some expression of sycosis; pains, rheumatism, gouty conditions, barometric sensitivity, aggravation from dampness and wet weather, eruptions upon the skin; in fact, if you study the history of the after-effects of gonorrhea upon the organism you will see much of it expressed in this remedy.

Subjective—Erysipelas usually beginning on the left side of the face, with great swelling, especially the eyes and ears; parts affected dark red, covered with yellow vesicles (Croton tig., Canth., Ran. bul., Pet.), with burning, tingling, itching, stinging, great restlessness and high fever, whole face swollen, eyes nearly closed; eyes puffed, swollen, hot, with tension and burning. Whole face, except forehead, greatly swollen; bright red, shiny, covered with vesicles; tongue, red tipped, dry; pains in the limbs, great restlessness and desire to change position frequently. Erysipelas bulbosus. Milk crust, thick crusts, with a secretion of fetid, bloody matter; forepart of head and side of face covered with thick, moist crusts, from under which an ichorous, often sanious, offensive discharge oozes; intolerable stinging, biting, itching, < towards night and by warmth. Fever blisters and crusts about the nose, red flush over the whole body, < in the afternoon; covered from head to feet with a very fine, red vesicular rash, which itches and burns intensely. Burning herpetic eruption; vesicles filled with yellow serum; clusters of vesicles about the corners of the mouth and lower lip (Nat. mur., colorless); salty, biting sensation. Large blisters containing yellow or straw-colored serum (Canth.), which rupture and dry into thin, brownish crusts; erythema of an erysipelatous nature with vesicles all over the surface. Erythema rapidly becoming vesicular, often becoming edematous. Scalp, abdomen, chest, lower extremities covered with a moist, itching, burning, stinging eruption. Herpes zoster with large, round or oval, yellow vesicles, with much itching and burning, with Rhus neuralgia, fever and restlessness. Backs of the hands covered with vesicles, hands hot, dry, skin hard, rhagades, Pimply-like rash with burning and itching; burning and itching pustules; urticaria from getting wet. Purpura, rheumatic, with shooting pains, restlessness, < in after part of night and better by motion. Carbuncles, bluish, gangrenous; warts, on the hands especially, large, jagged, often pedunculated with burning in them or a sensation of coldness. Scarlet fever, miliary rash, fever high, drowsiness and restlessness, tongue red, smooth, erysipelatous erythema of the skin. Variola, eruption sinks and turns livid; typhoid symptoms, variola, pustules turn black from an effusion of blood from within, diarrhœa, with dark, bloody stools. Chilblains, < wet or rainy weather, blue color of the part, much burning and itching (Agar.).

Subjective—Burning, stinging and intolerable itching. Stinging, corrosive itching, eczema or Rhus poisoning. Smarting and biting as of salt in eruption, < at night. Burning, itching tingling in eczema; the more they scratch the greater the desire increases, < warmth, warmth relieves almost every other condition in Rhus.

Burning, itching and stinging in tinea, alopecia circumscripta, tinea circinata, impetigo contagioso, hydroa.

Burning, itching and neuralgic pains in herpes zoster, burning and itching in vesicles, burning, < after scratching (smarting after scratching, Sulph.).

Aggravation—Rubbing affected parts increases eruption, < damp, wet weather; scratching, before a storm, night (after midnight, pains), perspiring, rest, wet applications.

Amelioration—Warm, dry weather, motion, change of position, heat, except itching. Wrapping up warm after perspiring, walking.

Temperament—Sang-motive.

RHUS VENENATA

Objective—Great swelling of face, head and hands with fever (Rhus tox.). Vesicular erysipelas of face and scalp, extending to ears, exuding a yellow, watery serum (Rhus tox.). White, fine rash under the skin, erythema

19

nodosum on right leg below the knee, erythema nodosum during an attack of typhoid fever, with pains in wrists and ankles, with an eruption of red spots, painful to touch. Large or small, clear, transparent vesicles scattered all over the body, with intense itching, not relieved by Rhus tox. internally; itching intolerable, proving by the author from handling the root; four cases of poisoning cured with the 40m. potency made from the same plants; vesicles much larger than Rhus tox., contents clear (Rhus tox., yellow or straw colored); Rhus rad., vessels large with tendency to ulcerate (Rhus tox., to form pustules). Ulcers having a dark blue blush on the arms and legs, sometimes phagedenic; it affects those parts more especially where the bones are directly covered with the cuticle. Ulceration of the lymphatic glands, lymphatic abscesses.

Subjective—Violent itching and burning of vesicles, blue clay applied locally relieved both itching and burning.

Aggravation—Touch. motion (reverse, Rhus tox.), rubbing.

Temperament—Sang-motive.

RUMEX CRISPUS

Objective—Contagious prurigo or army itch. Scabies (itch); vesicular eruption, < uncovered, cool air, Prairie itch, urticaria. Legs covered with fine, red pimples; eruptions from wearing flannel.

Subjective—Itching, pricking, stinging, < in the open air. Prairie itch, itching, < undressing, < in open air, from cold in general. Stinging in corns, itching deep in ears and anus. Itching in vesicles more of a pricking than a burning character; stinging, pricking, itching in prurigo. Vesicular eruption, itching only when uncovering or undressing.

Aggravation—Uncovering, undressing, cold air after scratching.

RUTA GRAVEOLENS

Objective—Acne rosacea, erysipelas of the forehead and hands, erysipelas after mechanical injuries (Arn.); smooth, flat warts on the inside of the palms of the hands, with sore pains. Fistulous ulcers on lower limbs. Skin becomes easily chafed from walking or riding, in children.

Subjective—Periosteal inflammation, periosteal pains and bone pains, < at night. Itching, > by scratching; itching of skin after meat eating; gnawing, jerking pains in ulcers. Bruised, lame sensation all over.

Temperament—Sang-motive.

SABADILLA

Objective—Parchment-like dryness of the skin, white blisters with red edges on right side of knee. Red spots on chest, arms, forearms, Thick, inflamed, crippled toe nails.

Subjective—Crawling, itching in anus (pin worms). Hot sensation in skin, burning, creeping, tingling, crawling as of ants.

Aggravation—During full moon, cold, cold air, rest.

Amelioration—Moving (Puls., Rhus), on getting warm, wrapped up.

Temperament—Sang-lymphatic.

SABINA

Objective—Black pores in the skin, especially of the face; acne punctata, boils on the buttocks, intertrigo and ulceration. Eczema usually dry until scratched, when it oozes a watery substance and again dries into a scurf.

Fig warts with intolerable itching and burning, exuberant granulations. Arthritis, gouty rheumatism, swelling, redness and stitching pains in the big toe. Ulcers, deep, with a thin scurf over them, much tenderness, < in the morning and evening, touch, warmth of bed, > in cold air and on elevating the limb affected.

Subjective—Drawing pains in joints, redness of joint, gout (Led.). Burning, violent itching and stinging.

Aggravation.—Pregnancy, touch, getting warm, in a warm room (Puls.).

Amelioration—In open air.

Temperament—Sang-lymphatic.

SAMBUCUS NIGRA

Objective—Bloatedness and dark red swelling, with much tension after contusions. Edematous swelling in various parts of the body, especially insteps, legs and feet. Edema, anasarca, general dropsy. Increased secretion of the skin and mucous membrane.

Subjective—Dry heat when asleep, profuse sweat while awake, hands and feet icy cold, the rest of the body warm (Cal. c., Sil.); night sweats, except on the head. After contusions dark red swelling, itching of scurfs on the head. Deadness, coldness, numbness in the middle tibia and feet.

Aggravation—;< after midnight, dry, cold air. Lying down, perspiring.

Amelioration—Pressure, bandaging, firmly.

SANGUINARIA

Objective—Circumscribed red cheeks, burning in the ears, with cough; under lip dry, swollen, blistered; blisters dry up and form crusts, which burn intensely. Ulceration of roots of nails (Sil., Hep., Kali sulph. Tub., Graph, Baryta carb., Magn. aust.). Ingrown toe-nails, unhealthy granulation, purulent discharge. Carbuncles, warts, fungous excrescences, roundish or oval, whitish patches on mucous membrane of nose, mouth, prepuce and anus. Eruption on the face of young women with menstrual troubles. Old, indolent ulcers, with callous borders and ichorous discharge, dirty granulations, dry, sharp cut edges.

Subjective—Burning of the soles of the feet and palms of the hands (climacteric or lung troubles), (Sulph., Phos., Opi.). Heat and great dryness of the skin. Pricking sensation as of warmth all over the body; in scarlatina it follows Belladonna; pains burnings.

Aggravation—Morning and evening.

Amelioration—Hard pressure, uncovering feet.

Temperament—Bil-vital.

SARRACENIA PURPUREA

Subjective—Erysipelatous swelling of the face. Miliary eruption on the face, with heat as if it were on fire. Scaly herpes on face and forehead. Phlyctenoid herpes, scrofulous eruptions; given in variola, it aborted the secondary fever in every case; eruption rapidly disappeared, dessicating without leaving pits; fever lessened, urine increased, constitutional symptoms rapidly subsided, there was no pitting; besides, the restlessness and sleeplessness was speedily relieved; confluent forms were much benefited by this remedy.

SARSAPARILLA

Objective—Moist eruptions on the scalp; pus from it excoriates parts passed over. Crusta lactea, when it begins as little pimples on the face, very itchy, forcing the child to scratch; eczema depending on a latent syphilitic basis.

20

Crusta serpiginosa, wildly spreading inflammatory affections of the skin; in open air crusts fall off and the new skin cracks; child very impatient. Falling out of the hair with great sensitiveness of the scalp when combing. Plica polonica, mercurio-syphilitic affections of the head. Face yellow, wrinkled, old, eruption-like milk crust, pimply eruptions on the face, eruption on the face with burning, becomes humid on scratching. Herpes on upper lip, herpes on the prepuce, moist eruptions about the genitals and thighs. Sycosis or mixed sycosis and old, dry sycotic warts, or syphilitic condylomata; squamous syphilitic eruption with bone pains. Rash as soon as he goes from a warm room into the cold air. Rhagades, deep and burning (Kali iod.). Herpetic ulcers, circular in form, with red, granulated bases, white borders, sanious reddish secretions; ulcers in the second stage of syphilis. Dry, itch-like eruptions with emaciation in syphilitic children (Iod., Syph., Kali iod.). Psoriasis, red spots after Mercury.

Subjective—Pain and burning in rhagades on fingers and hands. Scratching causes itching to begin in another place. Eczema, burning itching with chilliness, pains as from subcutaneous ulceration. Children have an old look, with dry, flabby skin (Baryta carb., Iod., Syph., Nat. mur., Opium, Kali iod.).

Aggravation—After abuse of Mercury, suppressed gonorrhea.

Temperament—Bil-motive.

SECALE CORNUTUM

Objective—Skin cold, dry, dingy, wrinkled, insensible, desquamating. Bloody blisters on the extremities. Boils, small, painful, with green contents, mature very slowly, and heal in the same manner; very debilitating. Carbuncles, extensive, dark, even black with much ecchymosis; purpura hæmorrhagica. Varicose ulcers with enlarged veins in old people. Ulcers turn black; indolent ulcer with ichorous, offensive pus, < by cold. General desquamation in scarlatina. Variola pustules of abnormal appearance, either filled with a bloody serum, or dry up soon. Indicated in feeble, cachectic, thin, scrawny women. Hæmorrhagic diathesis; small wounds bleeding for weeks (Phos.). Gangrene, dry form, especially fingers and toes; parts cold with loss of sensation. Cold gangrene of limbs, true anthrax.

Subjective—Limbs cold, with cold sweat, or with complete loss of sensation. Formication with a sensation of mice creeping under skin, crawling all over, under the skin. Violent crawling and pricking, jerking under the skin. Bloody blotches or pustules becoming gangrenous. Boils painful with green contents. Petechia with miliary eruption. Dry gangrene, parts cold, shrivelled, lead colored, with loss of sensibility.

Aggravation—From warmth and warm applications, external heat (gangrene).

Amelioration—Cold air uncovering, getting cold, rubbing.

Temperament—Bil-motive.

SELENIUM

Objective—Miliary eruption on the forearm, painful hang-nails; prolonged oozing from scratched parts; red rash on region of liver. Flat ulcers. Hair falls out on head, eyebrows, beard, when combing. Pimples or acne due to onanism. Face oily, greasy, shiny.

SEMPERVIVUM TECTORUM

Objective—Burns, corns, erysipelas, herpes zoster and

circinatus, stings of insects or rabid animals. Vesicles at the commissures of the lips.

Subjective—Burning in mouth, tongue, throat stomach, under the sternum. Burning vesicles, itching when touched.

SEPIA

Objective—Adapted to dark-haired people of rigid fibre, but gentle disposition (Puls.).; delicate skin, least injury tends to suppurate (Hep., Graph.); soreness of the skin, humid places in the bends of the elbows. Brown or claret-colored, tetter-like spots, (chloasma). Face puffed, pale or yellow, earthy colored. Yellow saddle across the nose, upper part of cheeks, yellowish brown or moth spots on face, around the mouth; circular spots on the face and under chin the size of a dime or larger. Herpes, scurf and black pores on the face. Dandruff in circles like "ring-worm"; eczema on the face, genitals, legs, bends of the extremities. Moist, scaly herpes, on the hands more particularly; dry, scaly scurf on the elbows, scald head, the eruption very moist and discharging a pus like matter. Brown spots, developing during pregnancy (during liver troubles, Lyc.). Ringworm-like eruptions every spring on different parts of the body, nettle rash on the face, arms, thorax, breaks out on exposure to open air, disappears in a warm room. Eruptions during pregnancy and nursing women. Acarus itch, suppurating pustules constantly renewing themselves; itch after the abuse of Sulphur, especially in women. Dry ringworm on the face; dry, offensive eruption on the vertex and back of head, itching and tingling, with cracks behind the ears. Pruritus during pregnancy, with vesicles on an acrid base on different parts of the body, hands, feet, armpits, vulva, anus, ears, hairy scalp. Ulcers, painless on joints and tips of fiugers, flat, with a bluish base, stinging and burning; warts on hands or neck with horny excrescences in their centre; small, itching, flat on hands and face; large hard, red warts, dark colored and painless. Varicose veins in pregnant women. Skin diseases developing in brunettes who suffer from chronic uterine troubles; reflex skin eruptions from uterine irritation.

Subjective—Empty, gone feeling in stomach, cold feeling on the vertex, feeling of weight on vertex. Urine scanty, reddish, with dark, coarse, sandy sediment, which adheres to the vessel; sense of weight or ball in rectum (uterine troubles). Skin burning, itching, or itching changing to burning. Itching in bends of elbows, tips of elbows, flexures of the body; eruptions often claret colored or brownish. Stinging burning in flat ulcers, itching in warts; psoriasis with vesicles; great uneasiness before strangers. Urticaria, burning, stinging, itching, < in open air. Itching often changes to burning when scratching. Itching of the scalp, behind the ears, face, margin of lids, flexures of the body, joints, external genitals, vertex, scalp in general.

Aggravation—During pregnancy while nursing, after scratching, riding in a carriage, during menstruation, sexual excesses, afternoon or evening, from cold air or dry, east wind, rest.

Amelioration—Violent exercise, warmth of bed, hot applications (Ars.).

Temperament—Bil-motive.

SILICEA

Objective—Light complexion, pale, dry skin, face pale, lax muscle. Tubercular or latent syphilitic patients. Controls suppurative processes (Hep., Mer.); yellowish color of the face. Lips, scabby eruptions, large, hard, brown crusts on the lips, blisters on the margin of the lips.

Cancer on the lip, itching, sometimes burning; border of ulcer red, with grayish base. Phlegmonous erysipelas; excessive, ichorous, offensive suppuration, dipping deep down into the tisues. Feet, foot sweat, offensive, making feet and toes sore, toes raw, or white and wrinkled, as if parboiled; perspiration horribly offensive (Baryta carb., Baryta iod., Psor.). In-grown toe nails, with boring, shooting pains, < damp or rainy weather or before a storm. Corns moist, between the toes, or on the toes anywhere; stitches in them, shooting pains in corns, < before a storm, corns become sore and tender before the approach of a storm. Nails crippled, grayish in color, horny, brittle, easily broken. (Graph.).

Bursæ about the wrists, with cold, sweaty palms, profuse sweat on the hands; hands and feet cold, perspiring profusely, yet the patient is not sensible of their coldness. Felons on the fingers, with lancinating pains. Burning stinging, aching in affected part; bone felons, deep seated; burning itching, aching in parts; whole finger is greatly swollen, bluish and painful to touch; run-rounds, ulceration about the nails, severe throbbing, twinging pains, with ichorous discharge, lassitude and depression. Caries of the bones, fistulous openings, discharging watery fluid. Burrowing abscesses in the skin. Veins smooth and shining, on the scalp; sebaceous cysts, pus scanty, smelling like herring brine. Synovial cysts, scirrhus of the mammæ, fistulous openings, discharge offensive, parts around hard, swollen, bluish red. Abscesses, boils, carbuncles, with fistulous openings, discharging a thin, watery, corrosive pus; pale people, with cold, clammy hands and feet; hard edged, fistulous ulcers, remaining after mammary abscesses. Inflammation of the breast; breast hard, swollen, deep red in centre, rose colored towards the periphery, sensitive to touch. Constant burning, which prevents sleep.

Subjective—Profuse perspiration of hands and feet, frequently with offensive, carrion-like odor. Hands and feet cold as ice to the touch. Boring, shooting pains. Burning stinging in cancer and ulcers. Itching and burning in eruptions; itching, biting after lying down, relieved by scratching. Shooting pains or stitches in corns and warts; ulcerative pains in ingrown toe nails, sometimes stinging pains. Intense burning at night in cancer.

Aggravation— < cold, sensitive to cold; night, uncovering.

Amelioration— < warmth, wrapping up warm, in a warm room.

Temperament—Sang-mental-motive.

SPONGIA

Objective—Goitre, red blotches on the skin, large blisters on the arm, herpes, miliary vesicles.

Subjective—Red, itching blotches on the skin. Burning itching, with desire to scratch; itching on skin, pricking, with fever, as if sweat would break out. First a creeping sensation in the skin, then the part becomes red and hot, followed by biting, itching. Measles, with dry, croupy, hoarse cough. Pruritus, biting itching. Fistulous openings in scrotum, discharge thick, whitish matter.

Temperament—Sang-vital.

STANNUM

Subjective—Itching, burning, pricking. Gnawing itching when undressing, burning in the hands. Tubercular affections, painful hang-nails.

STAPHISAGRIA

Objective—Anti-syphilitic diseases, eruptions, in patients who have had syphilis imperfectly cured. Skin dry, herpes about the joints, with crusts; nightly itching and burning; ulcers, in scurvy, mercurial and syphilitic patients. Fig warts, dry, pedunculated, after abuse of mercury. Eczema; yellow, acrid moisture oozes from under the crusts; upon denuded surfaces new vesicles form. Whole body covered with pustules, severe itching. Tetter on the hands, burning after scratching. Scorbutic ulcers, itching and burning ulcers, pus excessive, acrid, ichorous, fetid. Arthritic nodosities, periosteal inflammation (syphilis). Soft, humid excrescences on and behind the corona glandis. Large, easily bleeding lardaceous ulcers on the penis; condylomata about anus, like chronic eczema, with profuse discharge of offensive smelling serum. Lips full of ulcers and scurfs, with burning pains. Serpiginous ulcer, with excruciating pain.

Subjective—Burning when scratched; itching burning; itching, burning stinging as from nettles. Tearing, shooting, ulcerative pain in ulcers.

Aggravation—Night, anger, grief, loss of fluids from body, touch, sexual excesses.

Temperament—Bil-vital.

STILLINGIA

Objective—Pustular eruptions on the anus; scrofulous, venereal and other skin diseases. Secondary syphilitic diseases (Staph.). Chronic, indolent ulcers of the legs; periosteal nodes on tibia (Staph.).

Subjective—Excessive itching of the legs below the knees, < cold air, > warmth of bed.

STRAMONIUM

Objective—Skin hot, dry, flabby, dirty. Blisters and boils on the feet; eruptions, with swelling and inflammations; felons, when the pain is unbearable. Measles, scarlet fever, small-pox, in the febrile stages when there is violent delirium. *Red rash broke out when delirium ceased, perspiration accompanied the breaking out of the rash, fever and delirium subsided.* Petechia on face and neck. Measles, before the eruption appeared; great heat of the body with copious sweat; red, puffed face, much fear and anxiety, frightful imaginings, violent delirium; boiled lobster colored red rash in scarlatina, similar to Belladonna, but less redness, showing a disposition to suppressed eruptions, with fever and delirium. Sometimes the skin suddenly changes from a dark red to a brownish red or copper color, with intense itching. Abscesses, tumors with intolerable pain; old cicatrix very red; ulcers with thickened edges, sanious discharge.

Subjective—Face hot, red, with cold hands and feet, Tingling, creeping, crawling in the skin (fevers).

Aggravation—In the dark, when alone, swallowing, looking at bright objects.

Amelioration—Bright light, company, warmth.

Temperament—Sang-mental.

STRONTIANA CARBONICA

Objective—Sycotic eruptions on the face and other parts of the body; moist, itching and burning.

Subjective—Tension in the skin in various parts. Itching grows, < from scratching; when pain ceases itching begins, and *vice versa*. Rheumatic pains, < in evening and night.

Aggravation— < scratching, night, 3 A.M., uncovering.

Amelioration—Daytime, heat, covering up.

SULPHUR

Objective—Eruptions usually dry, whether herpetic,

papular, pustular or squamous and scanty secretion in the vesicular. Blotches in different parts of the body as from heat. Chapped skin, especially the hands. Chilblains, with redness, swelling and suppuration; skin thick, red on the fingers. Inflamed corns, dry, scaly eruptions. Eczema about the ears, margin of the hair (Nat., Ars.), legs, arms, genitals; pimply eczema, forming dry crusts bleeding easily; cracks, rhagades about the joints; skin all over the body dry, harsh, rough, pimply; no moisture, never perspires, always itchy, hands and feet dry, harsh, rough, never moist, as a rule. All symptoms dry and very itchy. Hands and feet burn at night, cold during the day. Herpes scabby and scurvy, scaly, rough, dry, harsh, < after bathing or after washing in water. Boils on the nates, extremities, axillæ, about the neck, dry, painful, very sore, with scanty discharge. Ulcers crusty, pulsating (Hep.); with raised, swollen edges, bleeding easily, surrounded with pimples (Hep.); tearing, stinging pains; discharge scanty, fetid pus; comedones, black pores on the skin, especially the face.

Eczema on the face, neck, arms, legs; yellow crusts thickly cover the diseased surface; fissures on the elbows, bleeding on scratching. Pustules on the hands and wrists; desquamating scales with much itching. Crops of crusts upon the scalp, arms, legs, since vaccination. Eruptions and sores upon the arms and chest, commencing as small vesicles, filled with serum, later on becoming pustular and forming into thick, dry crusts; itching very much when he gets warm. Varicose ulcers, bleed easily, secrete a fetid pus, burn and itch; after measles, scarlet fever, small-pox, suppressed eruptions in very psoric patients; recovery slow and imperfect. Adapted to very psoric people who are stoop shouldered, never perspire, sensitive to atmospheric changes, who are < standing, bathing, after suppressed eruptions.

Subjective—Itching all over body, painful after scratching; *itching, > after scratching but followed by smarting and burning*. Itching, < at night, in bed, covering up warm; obliged to scratch until it bleeds. Parts feel hot after scratching, formation over the whole skin; sticking pricking in the skin. After violent scratching, aching and numbness of the skin; voluptuous tingling itching, with burning soreness and smarting after scratching. Burning heat of the skin in fevers, feet; hands hot, burning; < at night when he first lies down; hot spot on top of head; body gets so warm must find a cool place or get up until he becomes cool (Mer.).

Aggravation—Evening, night, standing, getting warm, covering up warm, scratching, suppressed eruptions, before menstruation, bathing or washing, wet applications, rest, change of weather.

Amelioration—Dry, warm weather.

Temperament—Sang-mental-motive.

SULPHURIC ACID

Objective—Scars turn red and pain; blue spots like ecchymosis; purpura hæmorrhagica. Red, itching blotches on the skin, gangrenous tendency after bruises, in old people more especially. Hæmorrhages from all outlets of the body in exanthematous diseases. Boils, bruises, bed sores, contusions after Arnica; injuries from falling, chilblains. Red spots on different parts of the body, first red, then bluish, violet colored, then yellowish green after injuries. Easily excoriated when walking or riding. Erythema nodosum.

Subjective—Corrosive itching, burning itching; child has a sour odor from the body (Rheum); bruised pain, skin livid, profuse cold perspiration. Follows Ledum in ecchymosis; blood black.

Aggravation—After hæmorrhages, coffee and brandy drinking.

Temperament—Sanguine-phlegmatic.

SYPHILINUM

Objective—Eruption all over the body, not elevated. Can be felt by the hand on the skin. Pustular eruptions, discharging an ichorous liquid, and healing up, leaving a fresh, coppery pock mark; syphilitic rash, very prominent on forehead, chin, arms and front of throat. Abundance of fine desquamating scabs over the surface of the majority of the skin lesions. Secondary or tertiary eruptions of almost every form. Mild cases, or chronic cases not relieved by Mercury or the Iodides. Eruptions only slightly elevated, scaly; scales attached to their centers, dry grayish white, constantly falling off and reforming again. Eruptions of a dull, reddish, coppery color; seldom any pain, soreness or itching. Run-rounds, ulcerations of the nails of a syphilitic origin. Secondary syphilis in young children or infants; child looks prematurely old, skin wrinkled, puckered, bluish gray; child fretful, whining, cries faintly, skin full of pustules, macules or squamous eruptions. Hair falls out from any part of body in bunches or patches. Neglected, badly treated syphilitic ulcers.

Aggravation—Night, from dark to midnight. Summer, warmth in general.

Better during the day and cold

TARENTULA

Objective—Malignant ulcers and unhealthy skin;

anthrax and gangrene, with dreadful pains; boils, carbuncles, abscesses, when pains are extremely severe.

Subjective—Terrible pruritus; sensation as of an insect crawling; sensation as if insects or worms were boring or crawling. Pricking and itching over the whole body, hyperesthesia of the sexual organs, pruritus vulvæ. Burning, agonizing pain in anthrax, abscesses, furuncles. Great nervous restlessness and agitation, hysteric and choreic disturbances.

Aggravation—< walking, motion, contact, noise.

Amelioration—Open air, rubbing the affected parts, music.

Temperament—Nervo-bilious.

TELLURIUM

Objective—Ringworm on the face (barber's itch). Ringworm on any part of the body, < on the lower extremities; red pimples with minute vesicles on them (ringworm); herpetic circular spots, vesico-papular in form. Clusters of globular-shaped vesicles, half an inch in diameter, red in the centre of the circle. Herpes circinatus of the scalp, with constant itching. Fine vesicles on a slightly inflamed base on the nape of the neck and borders of the hair; disappears by desquamation of white scales. Body thickly covered with elevated rings of herpes, very marked on the lower limbs. Psoriasis in scaly rings.

Subjective—Intensely itching herpes. Itching worse at night, after going to bed. Itching, stinging, pricking, fine pricking stinging in herpes, came on like flea bites. Constant itching, night and day, more in the cool air. Alopecia circumscripta with intense itching.

Aggravation—< cool air, at night, sweating increases itching.

TEREBINTHINA

Objective—Passive hæmorrhages, purpura hæmorrhagica. Face earthy color, sunken, with exhaustion and debility; oozing of blood from mucous surfaces (Crocus). Lower limbs and abdomen covered with black and blue spots from a pin-head size to that of a pea. Hæmorrhages in fevers, thin, dark blood (Secale); erysipelas bullosum large, yellow vesicles with red areola, turning blue and black. Erythematous, scrofulous, even vesicular eruptions, similar to those produced by eating shell fish. Scarlatina with bloody, smoky urine. Chronic icterus; erythema resembling scarlet rash; intense redness, followed by vesication; vesicles filled with transparent lymph, with bloody urine, vesicles or blebs painful, with intense smarting and burning; affected skin peels off. Chronic, rheumatic and gouty patients; old people of sedentary habits who suffer with bladder troubles.

Subjective—Intense burning, soreness, smarting, itching. Burning pain in bullæ, or vesicles. Violent burning and cutting in the bladder. Tongue smooth, red, glossy, burning at the tip in exanthemata.

TARAXACUM

Objective—Unhealthy, pimply, sycotic skin. Eruption all over the body, itching severely, which appears to be a combination of lichen and urticaria. Pimples on the cheeks, wings of the nose, corners of the mouth with mapped tongue.

Subjective—Stinging itching.

Aggravation—While resting, fat food.

Amelioration—Walking, moving.

THUJA

Objective—Mental symptoms, loathing of life (Lac can.); very ill-humored and depressed, morose, shuns everybody (sycosis). Dry herpes on the head extending to eyebrows; dandruff, white, scaly, extending to temples and ears; hair falling out. Hair thin, grows slowly, splits. Eruption on the scalp moist, corroding on the occiput and temples, < from touch, > by scratching. Dry branny eruption on the eyelids, eyelash imperfect. Skin looks dirty, brown here and there, brownish, white spots, dirty brownish discolorations. Eruptions on covered parts. White, scaly, dry, measly or itching, crusty herpes. Pemphigus very painful. Chicken-pox (varicella). Small-pox; eruptions reached their height the eighth day; suppuration diminished, and pustules began to dry up, scaling off, leaving no pitting; variola, confluent on face; variola, pains in upper arms, fingers and hands, with fullness and soreness of throat; areola around pustules dark red, pustules flat, painful to touch, during the suppurative stage.

Wart-shaped excrescences size of a poppy seed on the hands; warts, condylomata about the anus, seedy warts, sometimes oozing moisture and bleeding easily; smooth, red excrescences behind the glans penis, warts all over the body after suppressed gonorrhea, more especially on the sexual organs, dry or moist, eruptions arising from vaccination, sycotic eruptions, moles, warts, spider spots. Erosions and rawness between the legs of a sycotic origin, constantly oozing moisture. Eczema of the genitals, red spots on the prepuce, changing to scurf or ulcer.

Ulcers flat, with bluish white floor, with indurated edges, surrounded with blisters, containing pus; deep, burning and fistulous, spongy on the edges; ulcers with serrated edges. Bleeding, fungus growths. Nevus of sycotic origin, moist mucous tubercles, washerwoman's eczema. Paresis, diarrhea, asthma, acute insanity, pustular eruptions, keratitis, ulcers, etc., after vaccination. People with dark hair, dark complexion, unhealthy skin, sycotic taint, either hereditary or acquired. Nails rigid, dry, crumbling, brittle, crippled, discolored.

Subjective—Trembling of the hands and feet, Biting itching in the skin, > by scratching, but continues to burn; sensation as if the skin was pricked with needles. Eruptions burn on applying cold water. Burning, biting on the scalp and margin of the lids in eczema; shooting in ulcers, dry heat of covered parts, when asleep. Perspiration on genitals and axillæ stains the linen yellow. Strong, sweetish, honey-like smell from genitals, fish brine odor from genitals (Medorrh.); sweats only on uncovered parts, when asleep, stops when awake (reverse of Samb.); profuse, sour smelling, fetid.

Aggravation—Night, heat of bed, at 3 P.M., cold, damp air; working, during menstruation, suppressed gonorrhea, after vaccination.

Amelioration—Drawing up of limbs, pressure.

Temperament—Sanguine-lymphatic.

TUBERCULINUM

Objective—This remedy, though very imperfectly proven, is rapidly becoming one of the foremost remedies in the cure of chronic diseases; it fills a place between Sulphur and Psorinum, and as soon as its symptomatology is better understood it will come into universal use. The mental symptoms are peculiar; the patient, although naturally of a kind and pleasant disposition, becomes sulky, snappish, fretful, irritable, morose, depressed and low spirited as the tubercular condition begins to develop in the organism. Tall, slim, flat-chested brunettes, who are weak and have a family history of tubercular affections, are the patients who receive the greatest benefit from this remedy; they take cold easily, without knowing how, emaciate continually, although eating well.

Objective—Soreness on the inside of the nose, with swelling and itching of the lips (rose cold). Inguinal or cervical glands enlarged and indurated. Hectic flush on the cheeks in lungs troubles; profuse nocturnal perspirations (incipient phthisis). Eruptions all over the body except the face and hands; eruptions in the form of blotches; ringworm of the scalp (Burnett); crops of small boils intensely painful, successively appear on the nose; *green, fetid pus* (Sec.), H. C. Allen's Materia Medica. Seborrheic eczema, hair matted together, offensive, bad smelling crusts, after Psorinum had failed. Tubercular forms of eczema, < on the scalp; lesions covered with bran-like scales (Syph.); itching, < at night, also worse undressing (Nat mur., Hep., Psor., Ars., Rumex). Tubercular ulcerations of a superficial character on forearm and tibia, chronic for years; pus scanty, greenish yellow, and of a pungent, musty odor. Acne of the face, forehead, neck, in tubercular patients, dry, of natural color of the skin; face looks greasy, pale, unhealthy looking, < during the menses (Nat. mur.). Ingrown toe nails; nails horny, hard, brittle (Sil., Graph.); tubercular inflammations of the nails, pustules on the hands with scanty, dark, greenish yellow pus. Skin pimply, pale, thin, anæmic looking, chilling easily and sensitive to cold. Ringworm; skin fiery red, much itching. < cool air.

Subjective—Symptoms ever changing (Puls.); takes cold easily, profuse, exhausting, pungent night sweats. Boils; intensely painful, green pus (Secale), emaciating although living well.

Aggravation— < in the night, itching, < undressing, cold air, damp climate, moisture, winter.

21

Amelioration—Summer, warm, high dry atmosphere, heat in general.

Temperament—Sang-phlegmatic.

URTICA URENS

Objective—Extremely distressing burning heat with formication, numbness and violent itching in skin of face, arms, shoulders and chest.

Nettle rash, raised, red blotches, with fine, stinging points, itching and burning as if scorched; requires constant rubbing. Eruption and itching disappears as soon as he lies down, and reappears after rising. Nettle rash coming on at a certain time every year. Vesicular erysipelas, erythema with burning and itching. Burns, when integument and the surrounding tissues are not destroyed. Rheumatism attending or alternating with nettle rash. Pruritus vulva, with stinging and burning and edema of the parts. Urticaria nodosa, on the hands and fingers. blotches red; itching on the hands and fingers; itching fever blisters on the lips. Lips, nose and ears swollen, eyelids closed and edematous, followed by small, transparent vesicles filled with serum, afterwards desquamating.

Subjective—Intense itching, burning stinging. Diseases that alternate with nettle rash.

Aggravation—< in the evening, every year at the same time, during pregnancy, after rheumatic pains.

Amelioration— > lying down.

VARIOLINUM

Objective—Small-pox, frequently indicated in the simple forms; removes quickly the dangerous symptoms. Dr. E. J. Kendall, of Detroit, Michigan, who has been in charge of small-pox hospital for the past two years, informs me that he has used this remedy more frequently than any other, especially in the initial stages of the disease; his observations were that it aborted many cases, and materially modified others; of course many other remedies were used, as the totality of the symptoms called for them. The death rate was probably the lowest on record in this hospital during that time, being only one or two cases out of over one hundred and fifty treated, which showed that true Homœopathy is far superior to any other system of medicine in the treatment of this disease. Drs. Swan, Blake, Kaczkowski and many others have testified to the virtue of this remedy in small-pox. It is said to change imperfect pustules into regular ones which soon after dry up; promotes suppuration on the third day, exsiccation on from the fifth to the ninth day, preventing scars. As a preventive to small-pox or a protection against it, it is far superior to the crude vaccine, and in a high potency is, of course, free from all septic infection, with no liability to the sequelæ that follow the vaccine of commerce. Probably no worse fate could befall a tubercular patient than to be vaccinated with the crude virus; there is no telling when the profound disturbance set up by the introduction of it into the system may end. Many forms of skin diseases and eruptions develop in tubercular patients after vaccination, as eczemas, pustular eruptions, moles, warts, besides nameless diseases outside of skin eruptions. Frequently it may be used in the treatment of such diseases, although the potentized vaccine is often a much better remedy for the bad effects of vaccination.

VACCININUM

Subjective—Mental symptoms, fear of death, nervous, impatient and irritable. Morbid fear of taking small-pox. Skin hot and dry with fever (Vario.); small pimples develop on defferent parts of the body, dark red, sensitive to touch. Eruptions of pustules with a dark red base, roundish, filled with greenish yellow pus. Petechia all over abdomen. Pains in the back, headache, fever and mild delirium before the appearance of the pustules. Pustules became very much inflamed, dark red, angry looking; ulcers dark red, erysipelatous, followed by sluffing; malignant looking pustules; high fever, face dark, dusky, comatose condition followed, and finally a complete coma and death. Pustules with dark brown, very thick crusts; dark, fiery red areola about it, very sensitive to touch; crust fell off in a week, leaving an angry ulcer, surrounding parts enormously swollen, dark red or of a dusky hue. Scar white, rough or smooth, depressed, like a syphilitic ulcer and later on became of a glistening white color. Scars break open every year at the same time he was vaccinated.

USTILAGO

Subjective—The whole skin is dry, hot and congested; copper colored spots on the skin like secondary syphilis. Scald head, two-thirds of the scalp a filthy mass of crusts and inflammatory products; loss of hair, with a watery serum oozing from scalp. Alopecia; complete loss of hair due to a long lasting congestion of the scalp. Boils very dry and hot. Painful destruction of the nails.

VERATRUM ALBUM

Objective—Skin blue, purple, cold, remaining in folds when pinched. Measles tardy in making their appearance; skin pale or livid; hemorrhages, but no relief, patient drowsy, weak, cold sweat on the forehead, threadlike pulse.

Scarlet rash in summer, eruption bluish, pulse feeble, burning heat of limbs, attended with coldness.

Ulcers bluish, hard, indurated, painless itching, but with a blue areola; pus scanty. Pimples in clusters here and there, thick rash on the face, dry herpes on the hands.

Subjective—Burning after scratching, heat and tingling all over, corrosive itching.

Aggravation—After scratching, cold nights following hot days in summer; perspiring after scratching.

Amelioration—After menses, rest.

Temperament—Bil-motive.

VERATRUM VIRIDE

Objective—Skin cold, clammy, bluish, insensible, shrivelled. Eruptions with intense fever. Erythema and vesiccation of the skin. Phlegmonous and vesicular eruptions. Scarlatina, with intense arterial congestion and brain complications; small-pox, before the eruption cerebral congestion and excessive nausea, vomiting and great prostration. Erysipelas; measles, with similar symptoms.

Subjective—Itching, tingling, pricking in the skin. Skin cold and clammy or hot and burning.

Temperament—Bil-motive.

VINCA MINOR

Objective—Crusta lactea, plica polonica, favus. Eczema or favus of the scalp, oozing moisture, hair falls out or white hair takes its place. Humid eruptions on the head with vermin, nightly itching with burning after scratching. Bald and face spots covered with white, dry, wooly hair, crusts on scalp.

Subjective—Burning after scratching, corrosive itching. Itching and biting on the scalp. Burning in ulcers, like bed sores.

WIESBADEN

Objective—Skin thick, like parchment; desquamation of the skin of the fingers and hands, preceded by pustules. Yellow spots on the face, cheeks, nose, upper lip, pustules appear and rupture, after which the yellow spots desquamate. Tetter-like eruption, with violent itching; pimples, vesicles, boils, mostly on the back; pock-like eruption extending over the whole body. Painful superficial abscesses. Free desquamation of the epidermis during perspiration. Cracks in the hardened skin of the heels and soles of the feet, desquamation of the skin about the finger nails.

Subjective—Uneasiness in the skin over the whole body, itching only when the skin is dry. Violent itching before the outbreak of perspiration. Biting itching as from salt, crawling and formication.

Aggravation—Before perspiration, when the skin is dry, < after sleep (Lach.).

Amelioration—Perspiring.

X-RAY

In dealing with the X-ray, either as a local or constitutional remedial agent, it should not be forgotten that we are dealing with a powerful force whose very name implies an unknown quantity requiring great skill and judgment in its use. It should also be remembered that the Roentgen ray is an intense ray from the chemical end of the solar spectrum which exists there in small quantities, and by artificial means it is produced and intensified thousands of times through the present modern generative process. Knowing this and having no present means to measure it we should be guarded in its use, especially in such diseases as tuberculosis, lupus, cancer, etc. To the follower of Hahnemann there is a deeper and more profound reason, when we take into consideration some of the fundamental principles of the law governing a cure of any disease. *One of the most vital of these principles is that disease must be cured from within outward and from above downwards.* We believe that there can be no other way to reach disease through the action of medicines but through the life force, and governed by this principle, all other means is antagonistic to the law; therefore, the so-called cures of skin lesions by a persistent use of the ray locally must be a suppression and not a cure, and we can safely prophesy that in time a history of such cases must reveal fully that fact.

The following diseases of the skin are said to be removed by the persistent use of the ray locally; eczema, psoriasis, lupus in its different forms, rosacea, tinea favosa and sycosis, erythema, epithelioma, and a number of diseases of the hair, besides the removal of superfluous hairs. Symptoms from a proving by a Brooklyn Hahnemannian union.

Skin symptoms. Absolute alcohol was exposed to the influence of the ray for some time from which the potency was made. Many of the provers were seriously affected by the proving.

A tendency to resurrect old symptoms or to reproduce suppressed eruptions, many of the symptoms were not heard from for twenty years.

Varicose veins inside of knees and legs with swelling and soreness. Palms of hands rough, sore, scaly (psoriasis palmaris); a number of cases cured. Tingling in skin as from electric shocks, with slight burning in nerve endings. Corns on feet become very sensitive and painful; thickening of the cuticle on soles of feet, smooth, red eruption on the face, < right side. Heat and swelling of the feet; tingling like pins and needles in left hand.

Rash on lower extremities with itching and pricking in the eruption. Itching, < getting warm. Discoloration of finger nails, falling out of the hair. Erythema bright red or bluish red, followed by vesication and ulceration; large blisters and blebs formed after its use locally with gangrenous sluffing. In the beginning there was no pain, when later on it burned like fire, an acrid thin coryza was a constant symptom in the proving, erysipelatous swelling on the face, eruption on forearm and hand like herpes, very sore to touch. Psoriasis of the palms, parts dry, rough, hard fissured, < by washing, cured with the c. m. The fetid odor in cancer of the breast was removed by a single dose of the c. m.; the case was past cure. A fan-shaped venereal wart was cured by the 1 m potency. A case of chronic itch suppressed by Sulphur was reproduced by a high potency of the remedy within a week.

The c. m., one powder daily, brought back in four days a suppressed foot sweat, fissures and bleeding of the fingers in a cook. Cured in a few days with a powder morning and evening.

Aggravation—< in bed, 4 A. M., bathing or washing the part in water, afternoon symptoms grew < (especially the pains), < perspiring, open air, > lying down warm room.

ZINCUM METALLICUM

Objective—Zinc has probably more pimply or papular eruptions than any other remedy, except it be Sulphur. Pimples on the forehead, back, face, upper lip. Pimples about the face in wine drinkers (Nux); clear water blisters or suppurating papules on the upper lip. Violent itching pimples on the chin; small pustules on the chin with itching; small, red, painfully sore pimples on the scrotum at root of hair. Small pimples, like boils, on the shoulders. Boils on the back and between the scapulæ. Rash-like eruption in the bend of elbow, papular eruption on the forearm, itching violently during the day. Large chilblains on the hands, swell, burn and itch violently. Bunions with stinging pains. Dry herpes over the whole body, suppurating herpes with lancinating pains. After disappearance of eruptions coma from cerebral exhaustion. Brain exhaustion after exanthemata; unable to develop an eruption; skin flabby, cold, child unconscious.

During measles took cold at the desquamative stage, followed by high fever, convulsions; urine scanty, brown, face edematous, convulsions following the disappearance of the eruption in scarlet fever, due to cold.

Subjective—Burning, formication and tingling between skin and flesh. Violent itching of the scrotum, < scratching. Small, itching points on the skin, sticking itching in a small spot. Violent itching with an urticaria-like eruption following the scratching. Painful, burning rhagades in the fingers. Sticking, pricking itching in the evening, <in bed; sudden itching here and there in small spots, < in the evening, disappearing immediately on being touched. Fine sticking itching over the whole body, with sour sweat, burning in tumors and in ulcers (Ars.).

Aggravation—Evening, wine, the abuse of.

ZINCUM OXIDATUM

Objective—Much used as a local measure to suppress numerous diseases or lesions of the skin. Boils first red and then blue, with hard areola and dirty yellow pus.

INDEX OF DISEASES OF THE SKIN

21

THERAPEUTIC INDEX

Abrotanum, **189**
Acetic acid, 189, **196,** 199
Aconite, 29, 35, 42, 50, 51, 56, 104, 189, 196, 231, 264
Arctium lappa, 184
Æsculus, **189**
Æthusa cynapium, **197**
Agaricus, 77, 108, 189, 227, **289**
Ailanthus, 29, 32, 189, **197**
Allium sativum, **197**
Alumina, 76, **197,** 241, 254
Ambra grisea, 198
Ammonium carb., 108, 190, **198,** 206, 233, 240, 245
Ammonium mur., 42, 78
Anacardium, 40, 76, **199,** 235
Anagallis arvenis, **200**
Angustura, **200**
Anthracinum, 57, 60, 62, **200,** 211, 229
Antimonium crud., 36, 45, 64, 146, **201**
Apis, 29, 32, 40, 42, 50, 54, 57, 60, 61, 62, 77, 105, 146, **201,** 209, 222, 231, 236, 265
Argentum nit., **202**
Arnica, 42, 50, 52, 54, 57, 104, 193, 198, **203,** 205, 208, 216, 245, 249, 260, 277, 291
Arsenicum, 29, 30, 33, 36, 40, 42, 50, 52, 54, 60, 62, 64, 68, 77, 89, 104, 116, 144, 183, 187, 193, 196, 197, 198, 201, **203,** 208, 210, 211,

220, 221, 227, 229, 231, 232, 234, 253, 254, 260, 264, 266, 274, 275, 277, 297, 309, 317
Arsenicum hydr., 89
Arsenicum iodide, **204,** 210, 231
Arum triphyllum, 32, **204**
Arundo maur., 190
Asafœtida, **205**
Astacus fluv., 190, **205**
Aurum met., 77, 146, **205**

Baptisia, 30, 40, 43, **206,** 242
Baryta carb., 64, 76, 78, 116, **206,** 239, 241, 260
Baryta iod., 260, 284
Belladonna, 29, 35, 40, 51, 52, 57, 60, 104, 108, 190, **206,** 242, 266, 272
Bellis per., 52, 233, 260
Benzoic acid, **207,** 260
Berberis vul., 33, **207**
Bismuth, **208**
Blatta orient,. 33
Boracic acid, 198, 207, 260
Borax, 52, 58, 78, **208**
Bovista, 78, 89, **209**
Bromium, **210**
Bryonia, 30, 33, 35, 40, 43, 51, 52, 54, 58, 59, 190, 197, 208, **210,** 212, 231, 234, 252, 264
Bufo, 60, **211**

Calcarea carb., 51, 52, 54, 59, 64,